General and Systematic Veterinary Bacteriology

General and Systematic Veterinary Bacteriology

Dr. (Mrs.) Varsha Sharma, Ph.D.
Professor and Head
Veterinary Microbiology, College of Veterinary
Science and Animal Husbandry, Jabalpur (M.P.)

Dr. (Mrs.) Anju Nayak
Associate Professor
Veterinary Microbiology, College of Veterinary
Science and Animal Husbandry, Jabalpur (M.P.)

Dr. (Mrs.) Joycee Jogi
Assistant Professor
Veterinary Microbiology, College of Veterinary
Science and Animal Husbandry, Jabalpur (M.P.)

Dr. Poonam Shakya
Assistant Professor
Department of Veterinary Microbiology
Veterinary College, Jabalpur

Dr. Ajay Rai
Assistant Professor
Department of Veterinary Microbiology, College of Veterinary
Science and Animal Husbandry, Jabalpur (M.P.)

SSPH

SATISH SERIAL PUBLISHING HOUSE
403, Express Tower, Commercial Complex
Azadpur, Delhi-110033 (India)
Phone : 011-27672852, Fax : 91-11-27672046
e-mail : info@satishserial.com, hkjain1975@yahoo.com
Website : www.satishserial.com

Published by :

SATISH SERIAL PUBLISHING HOUSE
403, Express Tower, Commercial Complex, Azadpur, Delhi-110033 (INDIA)
Phone : 011-27672852 Fax : 91-11-27672046
E-mail : info@satishserial.com, hkjain1975@yahoo.com

ISBN 978-93-88020-38-1

Composed, Designed & Printed in India

About the Authors

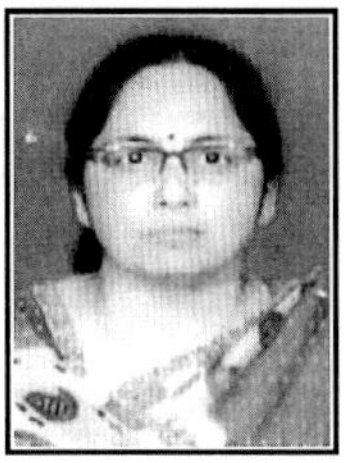

Dr. (Mrs.) Varsha Sharma Ph.D., is presently working as Professor and Head Veterinary Microbiology, College of Veterinary Science and Animal Husbandry, Jabalpur (M.P.). She has also served as Veterinary Assistant Surgeon in M.P. State Services for 4 years and 23 years experience in teaching, research and extension. Dr. Sharma has pursued her B.,V.Sc. & A.H. and M.V.Sc. & A.H. in Veterinary Microbiology from College of Veterinary Science and A.H., JNKVV, Jabalpur. She has guided several students in Microbiology from Veterinary and general stream of various universities. She has published about 01 Technical Bulletin , 03 Practical Manuals, 03 Review article, 75 Research article, about 115 abstracts and 25 popular articles and leaflets.

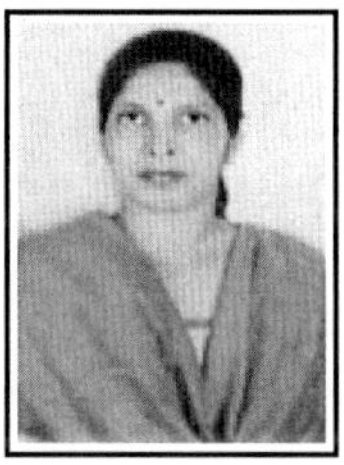

Dr. (Mrs.) Anju Nayak, is presently working as Associate Professor, Veterinary Microbiology, College of Veterinary Science and Animal Husbandry, Jabalpur (M.P.). She has a vast experience of veterinary extension, research and teaching. She is the recipient of University Gold Medal for undergraduate programme from I.G.K.V.V., Raipur (C.G.). She did her post graduation with specialization in Veterinary Immunology from Indian Veterinary Research Institute. She has pursued her Ph.D. from College of Veterinary Science and A.H., JNKVV, Jabalpur. She has a number of research and popular articles to her credit.

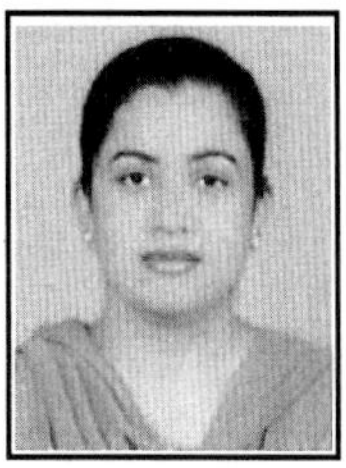

Dr. (Mrs.) Joycee Jogi, is at present working as Assistant Professor, Veterinary Microbiology, College of Veterinary Science and Animal Husbandry, Jabalpur (M.P.). She has secured 1st position in M.P.P.S.C. and served as Veterinary Assistant Surgeon in M.P. State Services for 6 years and has a teaching and research experience of about 6 years. She has done her B.V.Sc. & M.V. Sc. from College of Veterinary Science and Animal Husbandry, Anjora , I.G.K.V.V., Raipur. (C.G.). She has received a National Award and has a number of research and popular articles to her credit.

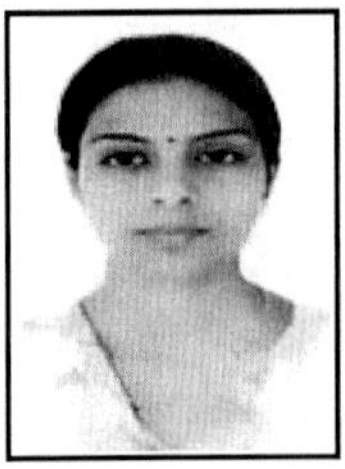

Dr. Poonam Shakya is working in the capacity of Assistant Professor in the Department of Veterinary Microbiology, Veterinary College, Jabalpur. She has completed her Bachelor's and Master's degree from Veterinary College, Mhow and grabbed the University Gold Medal. At present, she is pursuing her Ph.D. in Veterinary Microbiology, from Department of Veterinary Microbiology, Jabalpur. She has worked as Veterinary Assistant Surgeon for 4 years and holds 6 years experience in teaching and research. She has published a number of research articles in various national and international journals as well as popular and extension articles in magazines and newspapers.

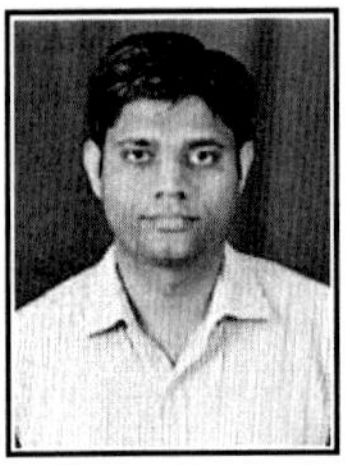

Dr. Ajay Rai has been working as Assistant Professor in the Department of Veterinary Microbiology, College of Veterinary Science and Animal Husbandry, Jabalpur (M.P.) since 2015. He has graduated from College of Veterinary Science and Animal Husbandry, Mhow (M.P.) in 2010. He has completed his Master's in Veterinary Bacteriology from Indian Veterinary Research Institute, Izatnagar, Bareilly (U.P.) in 2012. He holds 6 years experience in Research and Teaching. He has fellowships and number of research, review and popular articles to his credit.**1**

नानाजी देशमुख पशुचिकित्सा विज्ञान विश्वविद्यालय, जबलपुर
आई/4–आई 4 के, लाला लाजपत राय वार्ड (वार्ड 45), साउथ सिविल लाईन्स
जबलपुर 482001 (म.प्र.) भारत
Nanaji Deshmukh Veterinary Science University, Jabalpur
I/4 -I/4K, Lala Lajpat Rai Ward (Ward 45), South Civil Lines,
Jabalpur 482001, (M.P.) India
(Established by MP Act No. 16 of 2009)

प्रो. (डॉ.) प्रयाग दत्त जुयाल
कुलपति
Prof. (Dr.) Prayag Dutt Juyal
Vice Chanellor

Phone cum Fax : 0761-2678007 (O)
Mobile No.: 9522581917
Email: vcnduvs@gmail.com
website:www.ndvsu.org

FOREWORD

This is a matter of immense pleasure that Professor(s) of Department of Veterinary Microbiology, College of Veterinary Science and Animal Husbandry, Nanaji Deshmukh Veterinary Science University Jabalpur, Dr. Varsha Sharma, Dr. Anju Nayak, Dr. Joycee Jogi, Dr. Poonam Shakhya and Dr. Ajay Rai have published the scientific Manual on "General and Systematic Veterinary Bacteriology". This manual is based on new curriculum of VCI for student's benefits.

I hope that this manual would be very beneficial for undergraduate student to increase the scientific knowledge.

(P.D. Juyal)
Vice Chancellor
NDVSU, Jabalpur (MP)

Contents

Laboratory Rules

1. Attendance in laboratory is mandatory. Please be on time.
2. Wear a lab coat or apron-they are easier to sterilize than your clothing, if you spill a culture or staining reagents.
3. Be careful with Bunsen burners-keep them away from microscopes. Never leave the flame unattended.
4. No eating or drinking in lab.
5. Never lick your fingers, or put your fingers in your mouth. No mouth pipetting.
6. Treat every organism as a potential pathogen.
7. Consider all chemicals hazardous. Never taste any chemical or inhale any vapour.
8. Treat spilled cultures with disinfectant before cleaning them up.
9. Carry microscopes with two hands. Remember to wipe the oil off the lenses before putting the microscope away.
10. No radios, tape players, mobiles or CD players are allowed in the lab.
11. All cultures, whether in test tubes or petri plates, should be labelled with your name or initials, the date and the name of the organism. Plates can be written on directly-always on the bottom of the plate. Permanent markers designated only for laboratory use must be used to label cultures.
12. Most microbial cultures will be inoculated using a sterile loop or needle; once the transfer is complete the loop or needle should be sterilized again. Liquid cultures should be transferred using a sterile pipette and mechanical pipetting apparatus.
13. All test tubes should be placed in a rack before transporting them from one area of the lab to another. All lids on all test tubes must be secure.

14. All disposable microbiological waste should be discarded in the BIOHAZARD bag. Used test tubes should be placed in the designated pan to be autoclaved and cleaned. Used pipettes should be placed immediately in to the provided waste container. Do not place any hazardous or infectious materials in the regular trash. Do not place any hazardous or infectious materials in the sink.
15. Practice good aseptic technique by performing the following at the end of each lab exercise:
    a) Remove gloves inside out and place them in the biohazard bag.
    b) Remove lab coats or aprons, fold them inside out, and place them in the assigned drawer.
    c) Decontaminate your work bench by applying an antiseptic wash.
    d) Wash your hands thoroughly.
    e) Do not write in your lab manual or notebook until AFTER you have removed your gloves and apron and washed your hands.
17. Sterilize the inoculation loop before and after its use.
18. All reagents, stains and other equipments should be returned to their original place at the end of the laboratory period.
19. Unless otherwise directed all plates are to be inverted, all plugged tubes should have the plugs firmly set in to the tubes and all screw cap tubes should have the caps loosened one-half turn to permit gas exchange.

Classification of Laboratories

It is obvious that working with organisms in different risk groups requires different conditions for containment i.e. ensuring that organisms do not escape from their specimen or culture vessels or from the laboratory. The World Health Organization recommends three kinds or levels of laboratory:

1. Basic laboratory
2. Containment laboratory
3. Microbiological safety cabinets

1. Basic laboratory

This is the simplest kind. It is adequate for working with organisms in biosafety level 1 and 2. It should be clean and comfortable, provide enough space for the workload and the staff should have adequate sanitary facilities especially for hand washing and be equipped with an autoclave.

2. Containment laboratory

This is more sophisticated and is used for working with organisms in biosafety level 3. The principle is to remove from the basic laboratory those organisms and activities which are particularly hazardous because they are the most likely to infect by the airborne route, ingestion or injection of very small numbers. The object is to expose as few people as possible to the risk of infection.

The containment laboratory is, therefore, a separate room with controlled access by authorized staff only. It should be fitted with a microbiological safety cabinet. Its ventilation should be arranged so that air flows into it from other rooms or corridors and out to the atmosphere (e.g. through the filters of the safety cabinet) and never in the reverse direction. This will prevent infectious aerosols which might be released in the containment laboratory from escaping into other areas. Only highly skilled and experienced staff is allowed to work in these laboratories.

3. Microbiological safety cabinets

The microbiological safety cabinets provide a barrier between the worker and the infective material and are designed to prevent infection by splashing or aerosol. The air-borne particles are contained within the cabinet and filtered from the exhaust air through a HEPA filter.

Infectious waste disposal

A detailed information regarding infectious waste disposal is important to identify, segregate, transport and dispose off infectious wastes generated by laboratories, including those used for teaching. It also includes the disposal of unused and non-infectious sharp wastes generated within the laboratories.

I. Treatment of Wastes

1. Sharps: For example-hypodermic needles, glass, scalpel blades, lancets, etc. All sharps are hazardous because of the potential to cause cuts and punctures. They may also be contaminated with toxic or infectious materials which substantially increase the risk potential. They must be placed in a rigid, impact resistant, puncture proof and sealable container of appropriate size to protect handlers from being injured during collection and transport. They are disposed off through high temperature incineration.
2. Microbiological waste: General microbiology waste, once autoclaved, may be disposed off through the municipal waste collection system. Waste from infectious organisms, infected materials, imported organisms and genetically manipulated micro organisms are to be autoclaved and incinerated.
3. Media containing material of biological origin should be autoclaved or chemically disinfected (carbolic acid or similar disinfectant) prior to disposal. The media with growth should be collected in boiling water containing HCl acid. This is done to kill bacteria and HCl is used for hydrolysis of agar, if present in the medium. This treatment, however, is not sufficient and thus, material should be autoclaved for killing the resistant forms. After autoclaving the material can be safely disposed off.
4. Plastic wastes: Plastic wastes from laboratories may be contaminated with other materials. The disposal method for plastics must be determined by the nature of the contaminants. Normal laboratory plastic waste is autoclaved and disposed off through the municipal rubbish collection. Plastic wastes contaminated with pathogenic microbes, biologicals and Genetically Manipulated Organisms must be autoclaved and incinerated.

II. Storage containers

All laboratories must use standardised containers, bags and labelling:

1. Infectious wastes-Yellow bags with the internationally recognised biohazard symbol in black double bagging.

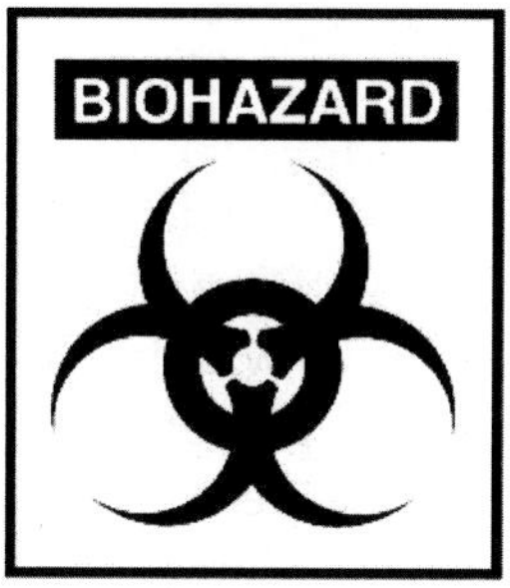

Biohazard Symbol

2. Cytotoxic wastes-Purple bags with the cytotoxic waste symbol (cell in telophase).

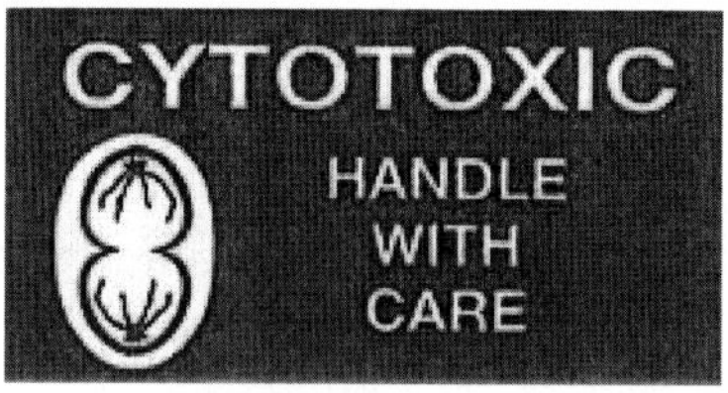

Cytotoxic Waste Symbol

3. Radioactive wastes-Red bags with the black internationally recognised radio-activity symbol.

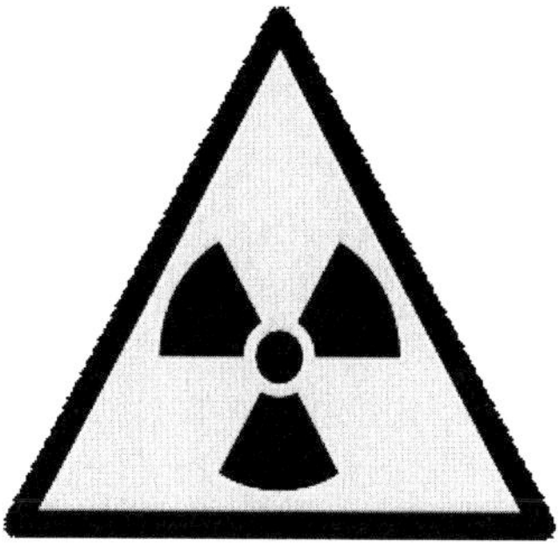

Radioactivity Symbol

III.Methods of disposal

1. Autoclaving : Used for the treatment of infectious wastes. An autoclave should not be packed tightly. There should be room for steam to circulate freely and to remove air which would otherwise depress the temperature even though the pressure readings are satisfactory.
2. Chemical disinfection : Used for mopping up spills and for disinfectant baths for routine laboratory work. Clear phenolics, hypochlorites, aldehydes and alcohol are commonly used for disinfection.
    a) Clear phenolics : These should be used at 2-5%v/v concentration. Dilutions should not be kept more than 24 hours. They are useful for laboratory discard jars and surfaces. These do not kill spores and non-enveloped viruses. Phenolics are not markedly inactivated by protein.
    b) Hypochlorites : Only products containing 100 ppm of chlorine are suitable for laboratory use. For pipettes, discard jars and surfaces, a dilution containing 2,500 ppm is adequate, but for blood spills and material containing much protein, 10,000 ppm should be used. Hypochlorites are effective against viruses as well as bacteria. They attack metals and should not be used on moving parts of centrifuges. Dilutions should not be kept for more than 24 hours.
    c) Aldehydes : Formaldehyde generated by heating formalin (liquid) is used mainly for decontaminating safety cabinets. These may also be used in the terminal disinfections of hospital premises.
    d) Alcohols : Ethanol and propanol at 70-80% v/v concentration in water, are useful for swabbing skin, surface and for standard clean up in microbiology laboratory. They do not kill spore but their activity is improved by mixing them with formalin or hypochlorites.

Transport of infectious substance

For the purpose of transport, infectious substances are defined as substances which are known or are reasonably expected to contain pathogens. Pathogens are defined as micro organisms (including bacteria, viruses, rickettsiae, parasites, fungi) and other agents, such as prions, which can cause disease in humans or animals. Infectious substances are divided into two categories:

1. Infectious substances, Category A- An Infectious substance which is transported in a form that, when exposure to it occurs, is capable of causing permanent disability, life-threatening or fatal disease in otherwise healthy humans or animals. For example:
   a) Infectious substances affecting humans-*Bacillus anthracis, Brucella abortus, Brucella melitensis, Brucella suis, Burkholderia mallei, Burkholderia pseudomallei, Chlamydia psittaci, Clostridium botulinum, Coxiella burnetii,* Dengue virus, Eastern equine encephalitis virus, *Escherichia coli* (Vero toxigenic cultures only), Ebola virus, *Francisella tularensis,* Hepatitis B virus, Highly pathogenic avian influenza virus, Marburg virus, Nipah virus, Japanese encephalitis virus, Kyasanur forest disease virus, Polio virus, Rabies virus, etc.
   b) Infectious substances affecting animals only-African swine fever virus, Velogenic Newcastle disease virus, Classical swine fever virus, Foot and Mouth disease (FMD) virus, Lumpy skin disease virus, *Mycoplasma mycoides* ,Peste des petits ruminants (PPR) virus, Rinderpest virus, etc.
2. Infectious substances, Category B-This category includes cultures, patient/animal specimens, biological products, genetically modified micro organisms and clinical wastes.

Packing of infectious substances

It includes the following packing:

a) Inner packaging
   i) Water tight primary receptacle.
   ii) Water tight secondary packaging
   iii) An absorbent material in sufficient quantity to absorb the entire contents placed between the primary receptacle and the secondary packaging.

b) A rigid outer packaging of adequate strength for its capacity, mass and intended use.

c) The packaging should be of good quality, strong enough to withstand the shocks and loadings normally encountered during transport. The packagings should be constructed and closed to prevent any loss of contents that might be caused under normal conditions of transport by vibration or by changes in temperature, humidity or pressure.

d) When transporting refrigerated or frozen specimens, ice or dry ice should be placed outside the secondary packagings.

e) Complete details regarding the infectious substance to be transported must be mentioned, such as type of material, date of collection, species, age, sex and breed of the animal from which sample is collected, name, address and contact number of the person responsible must be provided on the written document accompanying the package.

f) Lyophilized substances may also be carried in primary receptacles that are flame- sealed glass ampoules or rubber-stoppered glass vials fitted with metal seals.

g) If multiple fragile primary receptacles (such as test tubes containing cultures) are placed in a single secondary packaging, they shall be either individually wrapped or separated to prevent contact between them.

□□□

Exercise **1**

Orientation to Bacteriology Laboratory

Few equipments which are commonly used in a microbiology laboratory are described below:

Incubator : An incubator is a device used to grow and maintain microbiological cultures or cell cultures. It maintains optimal temperature, humidity and other conditions, such as the CO_2 and O_2 content of the atmosphere inside. They are essential for a lot of experimental work in cell biology, microbiology and molecular biology. The simplest incubators are insulated boxes with an adjustable heater, typically going upto 60 to 65°C, though some can go slightly higher. The most commonly used temperature for both bacteria as well as mammalian cells is approximately 37°C, as these organisms grow well under such conditions. Some organisms, such as budding yeasts, etc. may require an optimal temperature of 30°C. More elaborate incubators can also include the ability to lower the temperature, or the ability to control humidity or CO_2 levels. This is important in the cultivation of mammalian cells, where the relative humidity is typically >95% and a slightly acidic pH is achieved by maintaining a CO_2 level of 5%.

A simple bacteriological incubator is a double walled chamber, heated electrically. For adjusting and providing appropriate temperature, a knob with a calibration is present which maintains the thermostat system. The space between two walls is insulated to prevent any conduction of heat. A thermometer may be inserted from the top for noting down the temperature. The petri dishes are incubated in the inverted position; otherwise the water of condensation may fall and disturb the colony formation.

Water bath : A device for regulating the temperature of anything subjected to heat, by surrounding the vessel containing it with another vessel containing water which can be kept at a desired temperature. It is frequently used in a microbiology lab for a number of temperature related applications. Water baths are used to heat those substances, which can't be heated directly on Bunsen burner. However, only those materials can be heated with water bath whose boiling point is less than that of water. The temperature of the water bath is controlled by a thermostatic arrangement.

Centrifuge : A centrifuge is a piece of equipment, generally driven by an electric motor that puts on object in rotation around a fixed axis, applying a force perpendicular to the axis. The centrifuge works using the sedimentation principle, where the centripetal acceleration causes denser substances to separate out along the radial direction. By the same token lighter objects will tend to move to the top. It has a rotating unit, called the rotor, which has fixed holes drilled at an angle (to the vertical). Test tubes are placed in these slots and the motor is spun. The speed is measured in terms of revolutions per minute (RPM) and it can be read from the dial at the top. During placement of centrifuge tubes in slots, it is utmost essential to balance the opposite arms of the centrifuge. For this even if only one experimental tube is there, another is filled with equal volume of water and introduced right opposite to the experimental tube. The main purpose of centrifuge machine is to isolate and separate suspensions.

Colony counter : A colony counter is an instrument used to count colonies of bacteria or other micro organisms growing on an agar plate. It is a metal box with a transparent platform at the top placed in a slanting position. Inside the box a bulb is fitted to illuminate the petri dish from beneath. A magnifying glass is attached to the box above the platform which moves freely on the axis. It is used to magnify the petridish and colonies. The colonies are counted either manually or by using an electronic counter. More recent counters attempt to count the colonies electronically, by identifying individual areas of dark and light according to automatic or user-set thresholds, and counting the resulting contrasting spots.

pH meter : A pH meter is an electronic device used for measuring the pH (acidity or alkalinity) of a liquid. A typical pH meter consists of a special measuring probe (a glass electrode) connected to an electronic meter that measures and displays the pH reading. The probe is an essential part of a pH meter; it is a rod like structure usually made up of glass. At the bottom of the probe there is a bulb, the bulb is a sensitive part of a probe that contains the sensor. To measure the pH of a solution, the probe is dipped into the solution.

Water distillation apparatus : The water used in the preparation of media reagents, etc. should have neutral pH (7.0). It should be free from the interfering ions; tap water is not suitable for this purpose since it contains various interfering ions, such as sodium chloride calcium, magnesium, etc. Distillation plant is used to prepare distilled water- the purified form of tap water. It is practically free from the interfering ions.

In distillation apparatus, the heating coils heat tap water. When it boils, the vapours are formed. These vapours are collected in the condenser and are cooled by the circulated tap water. The condensed distilled water is free from the interfering ions and collected through the outlet.

This distillation apparatus is made up of glass. Heating tap water in a glass flask fitted with electrical elements carries out the distillation. The distilled water, thus, obtained by using this apparatus is called glass-distilled water and since it does not contain interfering substances it is used for preparation of culture media.

S.No.	Glassware/Equipment	Draw and write the use of Glassware / Equipment
1.	Test tube 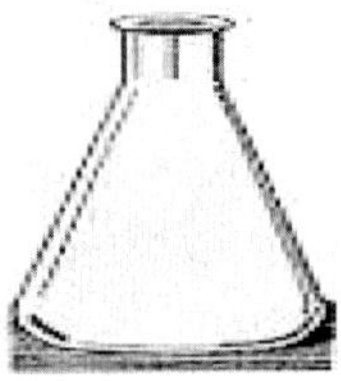	
2.	Conical flask/Erlenmeyer 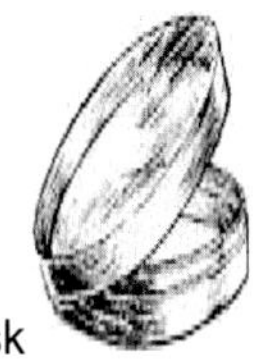 flask	
3.	Petri dish 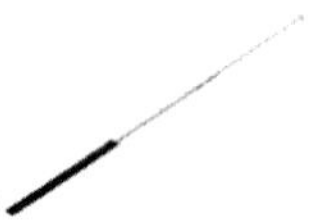	
4.	Inoculating loop 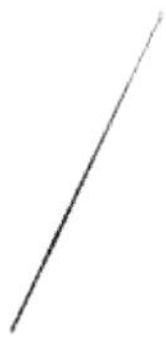 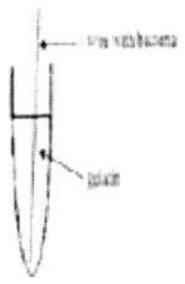	
5.	Straight wire 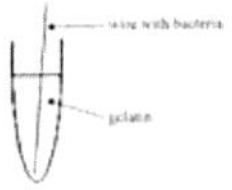	

6.	Spreader 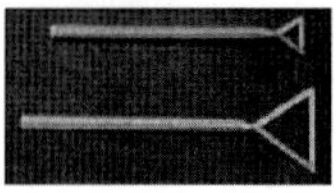	
7.	Forceps 	
8.	Glass pipette 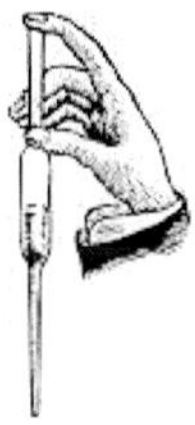 Micro pipette 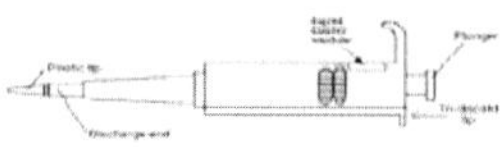	
9.	Rubber bulb 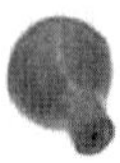 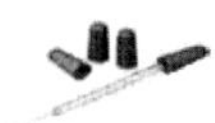	
10.	Marker pen 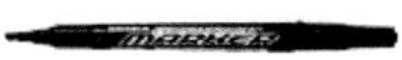	

11.	Apron/ Lab coat 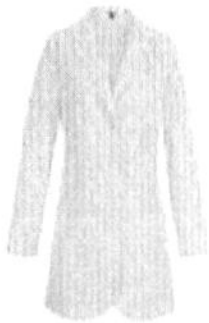	
12.	Bunsen burner 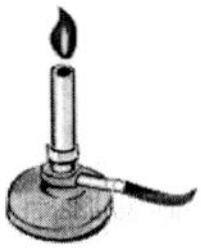	
13.	Autoclave 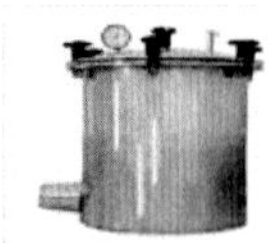	
14.	Hot air oven 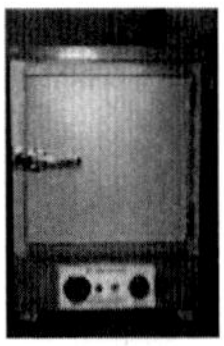	
15.	Incubator 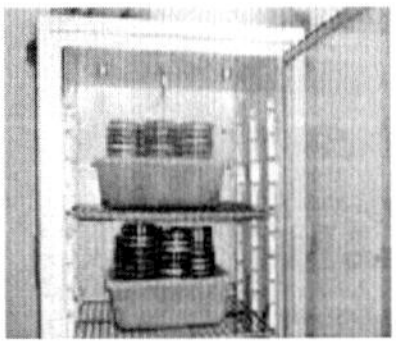	

16.	Water bath 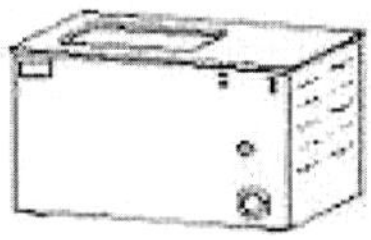	
17.	Thermometer 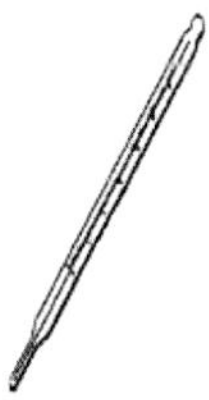	
18.	pH meter 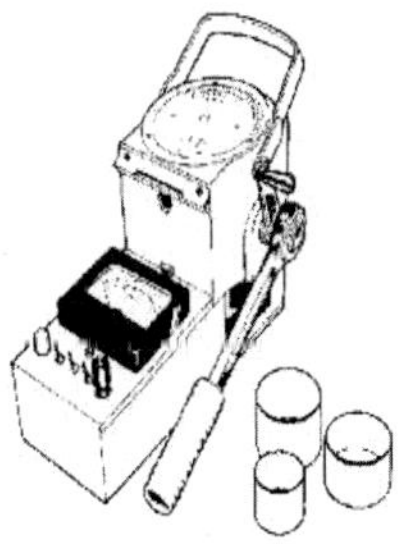	
19.	Refrigerator 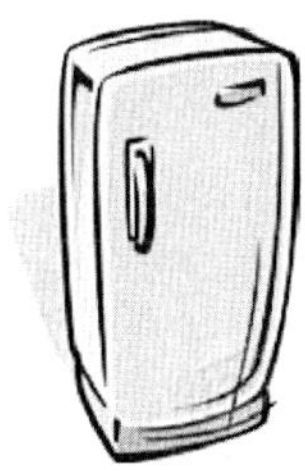	

20.	Mcintosh jar 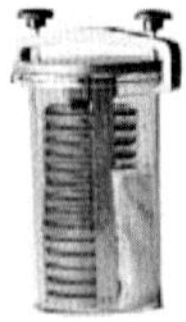	
21.	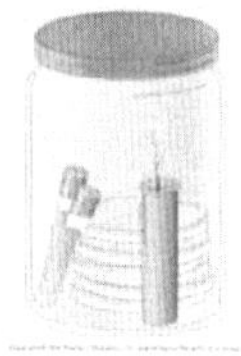 Candle Jar	
22.	Anaerobic gas pak jar 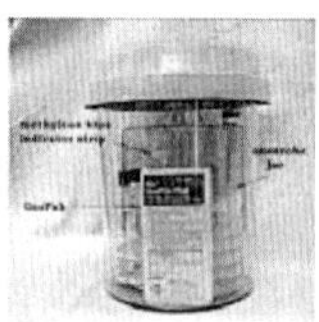	
23.	Beakers 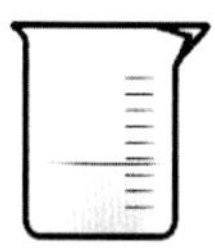	
24.	Flat bottom round flasks 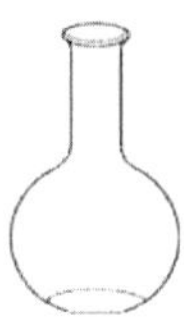	

25.	Measuring cylinder 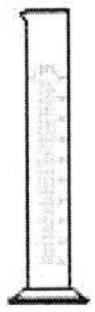	
26.	Drop bottles 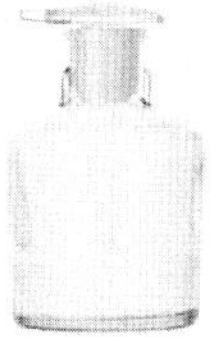	
27.	Centrifuge tubes 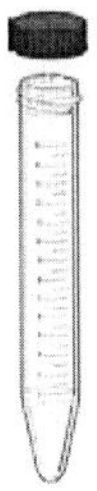	
28.	Cavity slide 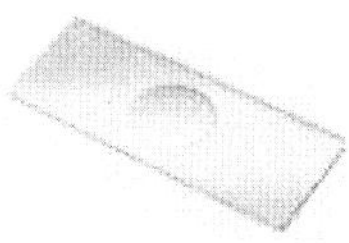	
29.	Tuberculin syringe 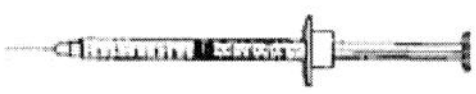	

30.	Microtiter Plates 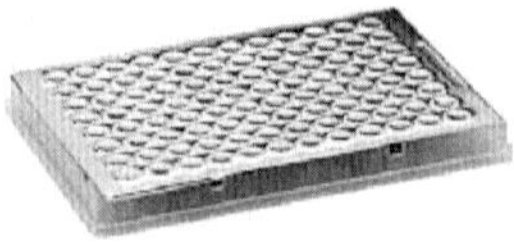	
31.	Centrifuge Machine 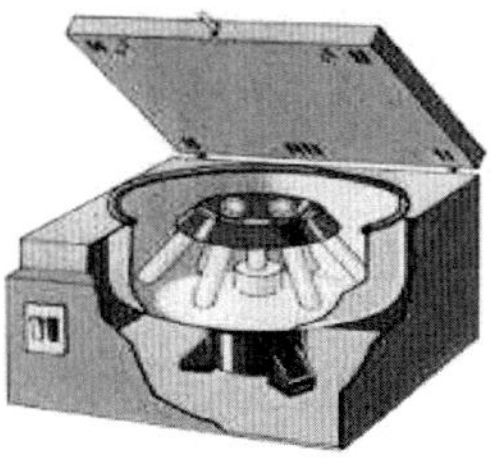	
32.	Bacterial Colony Counter 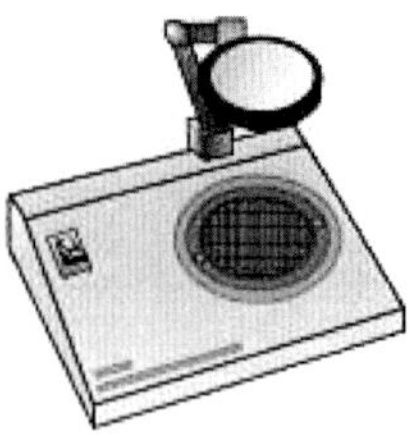	
33.	Water distillation apparatus 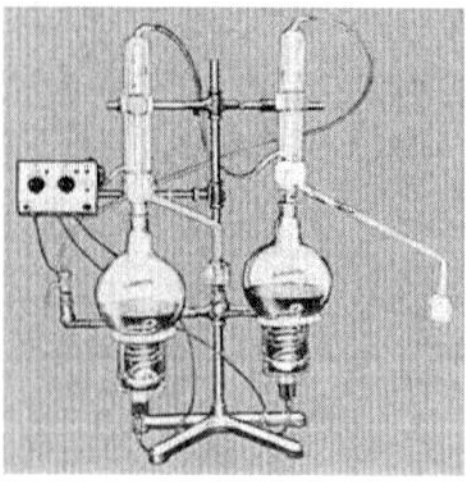	

34.	Sterile swabs 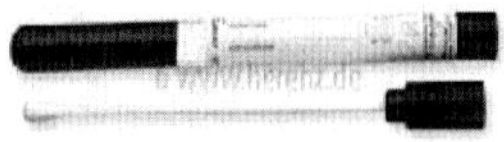	
35.	Teasing Needle 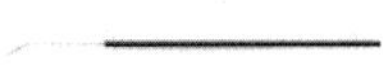	
36.	Instrument sterilizer 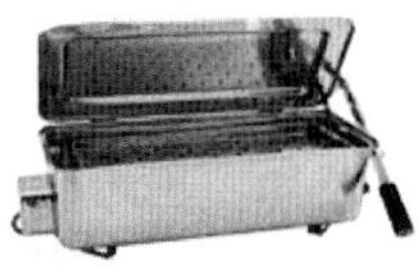	

Date: Signature of Instructor

❐❐❐

Exercise 2

Methods of Sterilization and Disinfection

The glassware being used in microbiology laboratory requires special attention. All microbial procedures essentially take place in glass wares. Hence, the glassware should be free of micro organisms and free of chemical substances that may hinder the growth or metabolic reactions of micro organisms under study.

The new glassware specially is given proper attention because it may contain spores of bacteria. The spores come from the straw and other packing materials. They may also contain some amount of alkali acquired during manufacture which hinders the growth of micro organisms. To remove alkali the new glassware should be soaked in 2-3 per cent HCl acid for 2-4 hours. This is called Neutralization. The acid is subsequently removed by KOH treatment.

The glassware that has been already used in laboratory should be made free of micro organisms. For this the medium is removed by autoclaving and the glassware is soaked in 3% Lysol solution for 10-12 hours. Subsequently glassware is dipped in boiling water, washed, dried, and then sterilized in hot air oven.

Sterilization

Sterilization means the complete destruction of all the micro organisms including spores, from an object or environment. It can be achieved by applying heat, chemicals, irradiation, high pressure and filtration or combinations thereof. It should be noted that sterility is a theoretical concept that can never be demonstrated with absolute certainty.

Methods of sterilization

I. **Heat :** It is the most generally applicable and reliable method of sterilization. It should be used, wherever possible. The living protoplasm of bacterial cells is composed of proteins distributed in a well balanced colloidal state. By applying heat severe imbalance, occur in the colloidal state of the protoplasm (coagulation of protein), which result in the eventual death of the cell.

II. **Dry heat :** It can be used to sterilize items, but as the heat takes much longer to be transferred to the organism, both the time and the temperature must usually be increased. The standard setting for a hot air oven is at least two hours at 160°C. Dry heat has the advantage that it can be used on powders and other heat-stable items that are adversely affected by steam. Dry heat is suitable for glass wares, such as test tubes, flasks, measuring cylinders, all-glass syringes, glass pipettes, metal instruments and paper-wrapped articles not spoiled by very high temperatures, as well as for water impermeable oils, waxes and powders. Following are the various methods of dry heat sterilization:

1. **Flaming :** It is done to inoculation loops and straight wires in microbiology labs. Leaving the loop in the flame of a burner until it glows red ensures that any infectious agent gets inactivated.
2. **Incineration :** It will also burn any organism to ash. It is used to sanitize medical and other biohazardous waste before it is discarded with non- hazardous waste.
3. Hot Air Oven.

Introduction

Hot air ovens are electrical devices used for sterilization of glasswares using dry heat. Generally, it requires a temperature of 160-180°C for 1-2 hours for proper sterilization of glass wares. Apart from glass wares, oil, powders, waxes, etc. can also be sterilized in hot air ovens. There is a thermostat controlling the temperature. These are digitally controlled to maintain the temperature. Their double walled insulation keeps the heat in, the inner layer being a poor conductor and outer layer being metallic. There is also an air filled space in between to aid insulation. An air circulating fan helps in uniform distribution of the heat. These are fitted with the adjustable wire mesh plated trays or aluminium trays.

Materials Required

Hot air oven, glass wares, non-absorbable cotton, paper or aluminium foil for wrapping, thread.

Method

1. Plug all test tubes and flasks with non-absorbable cotton and wrap all glass wares with paper or aluminium foil.
2. Arrange the material to be sterilized loosely and evenly on the racks of the oven allowing free circulation of air and thereby even heating of the load.
3. Switch ON the power supply and control the temperature of the oven by adjusting the thermostat.
4. Note the time when the desired temperature is reached (heating up time).
5. Hold the load in the oven at this temperature (holding time-2 hours at 160°C or 1 hour at 180°C).
6. Switch OFF the oven after prescribed time.

Precautions

1. Do not attempt to open the chamber door until the chamber and load have cooled to below 80°C. Glassware is liable to crack, if air is admitted suddenly while it is still very hot.
2. Do not over heat since it would char the cotton plugs and paper wrappings.

B. Moist Heat

i) **Steam sterilization :** A widely used method for heat sterilization is the autoclave. It uses steam heated to 121°C. To achieve sterility, a holding time of at least 15 minutes, and 15 lbs pressure is required. Proper autoclave treatment will inactivate all fungi, bacteria, viruses and also bacterial spores, which can be quite resistant. It will not necessarily eliminate all prions. Chemical or Biological indicators can be used to independently confirm autoclave performance. Most contain spores of the heat resistant microbe *Geobacillus stearothermophilus* (formerly *Bacillus stearothermophilus*), among the toughest organisms for an autoclave to destroy. For effective sterilization, steam needs to penetrate the autoclave load uniformly, so an autoclave must not be overcrowded. Moist heat is used for sterilizing media and other water containing materials in sealed bottles, laboratory discards and porous packaged material.

ii) **Autoclave :** An autoclave is a device used to sterilize media, plastic wares, etc. by subjecting them to high pressure saturated steam (15lbs) at 121°C for around 15-20 minutes. It was invented by Charles Chamberland in 1879. The name comes from Greek- auto, ultimately meaning self and Latin clavis meaning key- a self-locking device. An autoclave is a modified pressure cooker with a water heating device to produce steam.

Objectives

1. To become familiar with the working of an autoclave.
2. To sterilize plastic wares and bacteriological media in an autoclave.

Materials Required

Autoclave, plastic wares, media, water.

Method

1. Wrap all plastic wares with aluminium foil or paper.
2. Prepare the culture media by dissolving the dehydrated powdered media in distil water (as per the instructions mentioned for the preparation of media).
3. Ensure that there is sufficient water inside the chamber.
4. Load the autoclave and fasten the lids (diagonally) keeping the discharge valve open.
5. Switch ON the autoclave.
6. Allow the mixture of air and steam to pass out freely till all air has been discharged.
7. Close the discharge valve and let the steam pressure rise within the chamber till it attains a pressure of 15 lbs.
8. Hold on the pressure for 15-20 minutes.

9. Turn OFF the heat and let the autoclave cool.
10. Slowly open the air and steam discharge valve after the pressure gauge has reached zero.
11. Allow the material to cool before handling them.

Precautions

1. Never leave the autoclave unattended while the pressure is rising.
2. Fill liquid containers (such as containers containing culture media) only half full.
3. Leave space between items to allow steam circulation.
4. Always check the level of water in the autoclave. It should be always above the level of water heating rod.

iii) **Boiling :** Boiling in water for 15 minutes will kill most vegetative bacteria and inactivate viruses, but boiling is ineffective against prions and many bacterial and fungal spores; therefore boiling is unsuitable for sterilization. However, since it does kill most vegetative microbes and viruses, it is useful for reducing viable levels, if no better method is available.

iv) **Tyndallization (Fractional sterilization) :** It is named after John Tyndall. It is a lengthy process designed to reduce the level of activity of sporulating bacteria that are left by a simple boiling water method. The process involves boiling for a period (typically 20 minutes) at atmospheric pressure, cooling, incubating for a day, boiling, cooling, incubating for a day, boiling, cooling, incubating for a day, and finally boiling again. The three incubation periods are to allow heat-resistant spores surviving the previous boiling period to germinate to form the heat- sensitive vegetative (growing) stage, which can be killed by the next boiling step. This is effective because many spores are stimulated to grow by the heat shock. Tyndallization is, however, inefficient against prions.

II. Chemical sterilization

Chemicals are also used for sterilization. Although heating provides the most reliable way to rid objects of all transmissible agents, it is not always appropriate, because it will damage heat-sensitive materials, such as biological materials and many plastics. Some of the common chemicals used for sterilization are as follows:

1. **Ethylene oxide (C_2H_4O):** Ethylene oxide gas is commonly used to sterilize objects sensitive to temperatures greater than 60°C and/or radiation, such as plastics. Ethylene oxide treatment is generally carried out between 30°C and 60°C with relative humidity above 30% and a gas concentration between 200 and 800 mg/l and typically lasts for at least 3 hours. It kills all known viruses, bacteria and fungi; including bacterial spores.
2. **Nitrogen dioxide (NO_2):** It is a rapid and effective sterilant for use against a wide range of micro organisms, including common bacteria, viruses and spores. The mechanism for lethality is the degradation of DNA in the spore core through nitration of the phosphate backbone, which kills the exposed organism as it absorbs NO_2.
3. **Ozone:** It is used in industrial settings to sterilize water and air, as well as a disinfectant for surfaces. It has the benefit of being able to oxidize most organic matter. It is capable of destroying a wide range of pathogens, including prions.
4. **Bleach:** Chlorine bleach is another accepted liquid sterilizing agent. Household bleach consists of 5.25% sodium hypochlorite. It is usually diluted to 1/10 immediately before use; however, to kill *Mycobacterium tuberculosis* it should be diluted to only 1/5, and 1/2.5 to inactivate prions. Bleach will kill many organisms immediately, but for full sterilization it should be allowed to react for 20 minutes. Bleach will kill many, but not all spores.
5. **Glutaraldehyde and formaldehyde:** They are accepted liquid sterilizing agents, provided that the immersion time is sufficiently long. To kill all spores in a clear liquid can take upto 22 hours with glutaraldehyde and even longer with formaldehyde. Formaldehyde is also used as a gaseous sterilizing agent. Many vaccines, such as the original Salk polio vaccine, are sterilized with formaldehyde.
6. **Phthalaldehyde:** It is used in a 0.55%solution, and shows better mycobactericidal activity than glutaraldehyde. It is also effective against glutaraldehyde resistant spores.
7. **Hydrogen peroxide:** It is another chemical sterilizing agent. It is relatively non-toxic when diluted to low concentrations, such as

the familiar 3% retail solutions, although hydrogen peroxide is a dangerous oxidizer at high concentrations (>10%W/W). It is a strong oxidant and these oxidizing properties allow it to destroy a wide range of pathogens and it is used to sterilize heat or temperature sensitive articles, such as rigid endoscopes.

8. **Per acetic acid:** 0.2% is used to sterilize instruments.

9. **Silver:** Silver ions and silver compounds show a toxic effect on some bacteria, viruses, algae and fungi. Its germicidal effects kill many microbial organisms *in vitro*. e.g. Silver sulfadiazine cream is generally used for the antibacterial and antibiotic treatment of serious burns.

III. Radiation sterilization

It is used in the manufacture of sterile packaged products. e.g. Disposable plastic syringes. Some of the common methods of radiation sterilization are as follows:

1. **Ultra violet light:** UV light from a germicidal lamp is useful for sterilization of surfaces and some transparent objects. UV irradiation is routinely used to sterilize the interiors of biological safety cabinets between uses.

2. **Gamma rays:** They are very penetrating and are commonly used for sterilization of disposable medical equipment, such as syringes, needles, cannulas and IV sets, etc. The gamma radiation is emitted from a radio isotope (usually Cobalt-60 or Caesium-137).

3. **Electron beam processing:** It is also commonly used for sterilization. Higher dose rate and less exposure time are needed for sterilization.

4. **X-rays:** X-ray sterilization is electricity based process. High energy and high power X-rays are generated by an X-ray machine which are used for sterilization.

IV. Filtration

Fluids that would be damaged by heat (such as those containing proteins, urea, blood serum, sugar, etc.) irradiation or chemical sterilization, can be only sterilized by microfiltration using membrane filters. Membrane filters are commonly made up of cellulose. The filters remove bacteria by mechanically withholding them from passing through the minute pores either of the filter or by adsorption of the bacteria to the filter because of the difference in their electrical charges. This method is commonly used for heat labile pharmaceuticals and protein solutions. Usually a filter, with pore size 0.2 μm will effectively remove micro organisms. For filtration of other biologicals, viruses, etc. nanofilters with a smaller pore size of 20-50 nm are used. Biological safety cabinets are now-a-days, usually provided with laminar flows which contain HEPA (High Efficiency Particle Arrester) filters for maintaining a sterilized atmospheric environment in the cabinet.

Disinfection

Disinfectants are the substances that are applied to non-living objects to destroy micro organisms that are living on the objects. Disinfection does not necessarily kill all micro organisms, especially resistant bacteria spores; it is less effective than sterilization, which is an extreme physical and/or chemical process that kills all types of life. Disinfectants work by destroying the cell wall of microbes or interfering with the metaboloism. Sanitizers are substances that simultaneously clean and disinfect. Disinfectants are frequently used in laboratories, hospitals, kitchens and bathrooms to kill infectious organisms.

Properties of disinfectants

1. A perfect disinfectant should offer complete and full microbiological sterilization.
2. It should not harm humans and other useful forms of life.
3. It should be inexpensive.
4. It should be non-corrosive.
5. It should be fast acting even in the presence of organic substances, such as those in body fluid.
6. It should easily penetrate material to be disinfected without damaging or discolouring the materials.
7. It should be easy to prepare and stable even when exposed to light, heat, or other environmental factors.
8. It should be easy to obtain and use.
9. It should not have an unpleasant odour.

The choice of disinfectant to be used depends on the particular situation. Some disinfectants have a wide spectrum (kill many different types of micro organisms), while others kill a smaller range of disease causing organisms but are preferred for other properties (they may be non-corrosive, non-toxic, or inexpensive). Bacteria can increase in number very quickly, which enables them to evolve rapidly. Should some bacteria survive a chemical attack they give rise to new generations composed completely of bacteria that have resistance to the particular chemical used. Under a sustained chemical attack, the surviving bacteria in successive generations are increasingly resistant to the chemical used, and ultimately the chemical is rendered ineffective.

Types of disinfectants

1. **Air disinfectants:** They are typically chemical substances capable of disinfecting micro organisms suspended in the air. An air disinfectant must be dispersed either as an **aerosol** or **vapour** at a sufficient concentration in the air to cause the number of viable infectious micro organisms to be significantly reduced. Example: Glycols.
2. **Alcohols:** Alcohols, usually ethanol or isopropanol, are sometimes used as a disinfectant, but more often as an antiseptic (the distinction being that alcohol tends to be used on living tissue rather than non-living surfaces).
3. **Aldehydes:** Aldehydes, such as formaldehyde and glutaraldehyde have a wide microbicidal activity and are sporicidal and fungicidal.
4. **Oxidizing agents:** They act by oxidizing the cell membrane of micro organisms, which results in a loss of structure and leads to cell lysis and death. Example: chlorine and oxygen.
    a) **Sodium hypochlorite:** Commonly used household bleach to disinfect drains, toilets, and other surfaces.
    b) **Hydrogen peroxide:** It is used in laboratories and hospitals to disinfect surfaces.
    c) **Hydrogen peroxide vapour:** It is used as a medical sterilant and as room disinfectant. Vaporized hydrogen peroxide is one of the chemicals approved for decontamination of anthrax spores from contaminated buildings. It has also been shown

to be effective in removing exotic animal viruses, such as avian influenza and Newcastle disease from equipment and surfaces.

d) **Iodine:** Iodine is usually dissolved in an organic solvent or as Lugol's iodine solution. It is used in the poultry industry. It is added to the birds drinking water. In human and veterinary medicine, iodine products are widely used to prepare incision sites prior to surgery. Although it increases both scar tissue formation and healing time, tincture of iodine is used as an antiseptic for skin cuts and scrapes, and remains among the most effective antiseptics known.

e) **Ozone:** It is a gas used for disinfecting water, laundry, foods, air, and surfaces.

f) **Potassium permanganate ($KMnO_4$):** It is a purplish black crystalline powder that colours everything it touches, through a strong oxidizing action. It is widely used in swimming pools, to disinfect community water ponds and wells and also to wounds in dilute solutions.

g) **Potassium peroxymonosulphate:** It is a wide spectrum disinfectant used in laboratories. It kills bacteria, viruses and fungi.

5. **Phenolics:** They are active ingredients in some household disinfectants. They are also found in some mouth washes and in disinfectant soap and hand washes. Example: Phenol (oldest known disinfectant used by Lister), Chloroxylenol (principal ingredient in Dettol), etc.

6. **Quaternary ammonium compounds:** Such as benzalkonium chloride are used against bacteria, enveloped viruses, pathogenic fungi and mycobacteria.

7. **Silver:** It has antimicrobial properties. Silver dihydrogen citrate (SDC) is a chelated form of silver which kill micro organisms by two modes of action:

   i) The silver ions deactivates structural and metabolic membrane proteins, leading to microbial death.

   ii) The microbes view SDC as a food source, allowing the silver ion to enter the microbe. Once inside the organism, the silver ion denatures the DNA, which halts the microbe's ability to replicate, leading to its death.

Questions

Q1. Name the materials which can be sterilized in a hot air oven.

Q2. Which form of heat is used in hot air oven for sterilization?

Q3. Mention the temperature and time specifications required for sterilization in a hot air oven.

Q4. What is the principle of autoclave?

Q5. Name the materials which can be sterilized in an autoclave.

Q6. Which form of heat is used for sterilization in an autoclave?

Q7. Mention the temperature, pressure and time specifications for sterilization in an autoclave.

Date: Signature of Instructor

Aseptic Techniques

Objectives

1. To learn aseptic techniques for working with bacterial cultures.

Micro organisms include bacteria, fungi and molds, and they are everywhere—in the air, in water, and on every kind of surface imaginable. Their widespread presence means that microbiologists have to take certain precautions, when working with bacteria to avoid contamination. When studying bacteria, it is important that the bacterial culture be pure, meaning that it contains only cells of that bacterial species. Otherwise, the results of any tests or procedures are meaningless. From a clinical standpoint, it is imperative to avoid cross-contamination of samples, lest the wrong diagnosis be made.

The frequently used aseptic techniques include - transferring broth culture to broth, slant culture to broth, broth culture to slant, and slant culture to plate culture.

Materials Required

Test tube rack, 15 ml nutrient broth culture of bacteria, 1 nutrient agar slant culture of bacteria, 2-5 ml tubes of sterile nutrient broth, 1 nutrient agar plate, inoculating loop.

Procedure

I. Transfer of bacteria from broth to broth

1. Light your Bunsen burner.
2. Sterilize your loop by holding it in the flame of the Bunsen burner until it glows red
3. Let the loop cool thoroughly.
4. With the loop in your dominant hand, pick up the broth culture in the other hand and shake it gently to make sure it's mixed.
5. With the little finger of the hand holding the loop, grasp the cap/cotton of the tube and pull it off.
6. Immediately flame the mouth of the tube. Remove the tube from the flame.

7. Insert the loop into the culture, making sure you don't go too deep and risk exposing the culture to an unflamed portion of your loop.
8. Remove the loop, flame the mouth of the culture, and replace the cap/cotton. Set the tube down in the rack.
9. Pick up the new tube of sterile broth, remove the cap as before, and flame the mouth of the tube.
10. Without flaming the loop, insert the loop containing some of the original culture into the new tube. Remove the loop and flame the mouth of the tube before replacing the cap/cotton.
11. Flame the loop to sterilize it.

II. Transfer of bacteria from agar to broth

1. With a loop sterilized and cooled as described in Part 1 in one hand, pick up your agar slant culture of bacteria in the other. Remove the cap/cotton as before, and flame the mouth of the tube.
2. Insert the loop and pick up a small amount of bacterial growth. Remove the loop, flame the mouth of the tube, and replace the cap/cotton. Put the culture back in your rack.
3. Pick up a fresh tube of nutrient broth, remove the cap/cotton, and flame the mouth of the tube.
4. Insert the loop containing the bacteria from the slant culture and stir gently to dislodge the bacteria into the broth.
5. Remove the loop, flame the mouth of the tube, replace the cap/ cotton, and set it in your rack.
6. Sterilize your loop.

III. Transfer of bacteria from broth to agar

1. With a loop sterilized and cooled as described above, pick up your broth culture of bacteria. Remove the cap/cotton as before, and flame the mouth of the tube.
2. Insert the loop to get a drop of culture. Remove the loop, flame the mouth of the tube, and replace the cap/cotton. Put the culture back in your rack.

3. Carefully lift the lid of your agar plate with the hand that is not holding the loop. Do NOT set the lid down anywhere at any time.
4. Carefully streak the loop back and forth over the surface of the plate.
5. Put the lid back down and flame your loop.
6. Incubate all inoculated cultures in incubator at 37°C at least for 24-48 hours and then record your observations.

Result & Observations

Q1. Did something grow in all of your transfers? If not, what could have been the problem?

Q2. Do any of your agar plates appear to be contaminated?

Q3. How would you know if your broth cultures were contaminated with a microbe other than the one you wanted to grow?

Date: Signature of Instructor

❑❑❑

Exercise 3

Preparation of Culture Media for Cultivation of Aerobic and Anaerobic Bacteria

Objectives

1. To be familiar with different types of culture media used in a microbiology laboratory.
2. To prepare different culture media.

Introduction

Micro organisms need nutrients, a source of energy and certain environmental conditions in order to grow and reproduce. In the environment, microbes have adapted to the habitats most suitable for their needs, in the laboratory, however, these requirements must be met by a culture medium. The media that are used in the microbiology laboratories to culture bacteria are referred to as *artificial* or *synthetic* media because they do not occur naturally; rather, they are prepared in the lab. These media contains nutrients to grow organisms outside of their natural habitats. It can be used to:

1. Enrich the numbers of bacteria.
2. Select for certain bacteria and suppress others.
3. Differentiate among different kinds of bacteria.

Classification of media: Culture media can be classified by consistency as:

1. Liquid- also known as broth. e.g. Peptone water, Nutrient broth.
2. Solid- made by adding agar (1-2%) to liquid media. e.g. Nutrient agar.

3. Semi solid- made by adding agar (0.6%) to liquid medium. e.g. Hugh and Leifson media (Oxidation fermentation media).

Culture media can also be classified as the following:

1. Basic Media : These are simple media, such as nutrient agar, nutrient broth and peptone water that will support the growth of micro-organisms that don't have special nutritional requirement. They are often used in the preparation of enriched media.
2. Enriched Media : An enriched media is a broth or solid medium containing a rich supply of special nutrients (e.g. Blood, serum or egg) that promotes the growth of fastidious organisms. It is made by adding extra nutrients to a nutrient agar (basic medium). Commonly used examples are Blood agar and Chocolate agar, both of which are rich in nutrients and free from inhibitory substances.
3. Selective Media : These media contain substances (e.g. bile salt or other chemicals, dyes, antibiotics) which inhibit the growth of one organism to allow the growth of another to be more clearly demonstrated e.g. XLD (Xylose Lysine Deoxycholate Agar) and DCA (Desoxycholate Citrate Agar) are used for the isolation of Salmonella and Shigella species.
4. Differential (Indicator) Media : These media contain a substance that is changed visibly as a result of the metabolism of particular organism e.g. Keigler Iron Agar (KIA) and Triple Sugar Iron Agar (TSI), both differentiate between different types of Enterobacteriaceae on the basis of their ability to ferment carbohydrates.
5. Selective and Differential Media : An example of this is MacConkey Agar which is selective for enteric and other Gram-negative bacteria while inhibits gram-positive bacteria, and has an indicator (neutral red) to differentiate between ***lactose*** and ***non-lactose*** fermenting organisms. Another example, *MSA (Mannitol Salt Agar)* is selective and differential to grow *Staphylococcus aureus.*

Materials Required

Dehydrated media powder, weighing balance, conical flask, measuring cylinder, distilled water, cotton wool, autoclave, sterilized plates/test tubes.

Procedure

1. Read the label on the powdered media for instructions, on how to use, before preparation of the media.
2. Rinse all glassware in sterile distilled water before using.
3. Weigh out the correct amount of media to be used, using balance.
4. Pour the weighed out media into a flask and add distilled water with vigorous swirling to achieve an even suspension.
5. Cover the top of the flask with a cotton plug.
6. Place the flask into the autoclave and start the sterilization procedure.
7. After sterilization remove the flask from autoclave and cool it to about 55°C temperature.
8. Pour the sterilized media to sterile plates/test tubes.
9. Let the media solidify.
10. Keep the plates in incubator overnight for sterility check.
11. Remove plates from incubator next day.
12. Store at 4°C temperature in refrigerator for future use.

Precautions

1. Weigh the dehydrated media contents accurately.
2. Close the media bottle tightly after use as the dehydrated media is usually hygroscopic.
3. Pour the media in plates/test tubes at appropriate temperature.
4. Avoid the presence of air bubbles in media.

Observation

Examine the media plates/test tubes prepared and record your observations.

Result

Questions

Q1. Is the sterilized media sterile after incubation? Explain.

Q2. Why are the petri plates kept in an inverted position?

Date: Signature of Instructor

❑❑❑

Exercise **4**

Isolation of Bacteria in Pure Culture and Methods of Inoculation

A) Streak Plate Method

The purpose of this experiment is to separate a mixed bacterial culture to obtain single, isolated colonies of each bacterial species. When working with micro-organisms, it is desirable to start with single, isolated colonies to ensure you are working with a pure culture. Cultures that are visible on the surface of solid media are called colonies. A colony forms on a plate when a single microbe is inoculated onto the surface of the plate and reproduces until there are enough cells to form a visible colony. Since a colony theoretically forms from a single cell, a colony should then represent a pure culture. One way to obtain single, isolated colonies is using the Streak Plate method.

Objectives

The streaking procedure is used in order to check:

1. Whether a culture consists of only one organism (a "pure culture") or if there are more than one organisms in it (contaminated).
2. Whether a culture is viable, i.e., able to grow (perhaps a "stock" culture kept for some time in the refrigerator).

Principle

Individual microbial cells can be separated by dragging them over the surface of the agar, and then given a chance to grow into individual colonies.

Materials Required

Petri dish containing (set-fairly firm-dry) nutrient agar, wire loops, mounted in metal handle, inoculum material in broth or other (liquid) medium.

Procedure

1. Clean an area of bench (table top) and wipe it with disinfectant.
2. Flame a wire loop, bring it to red heat and leave it for few seconds to cool.

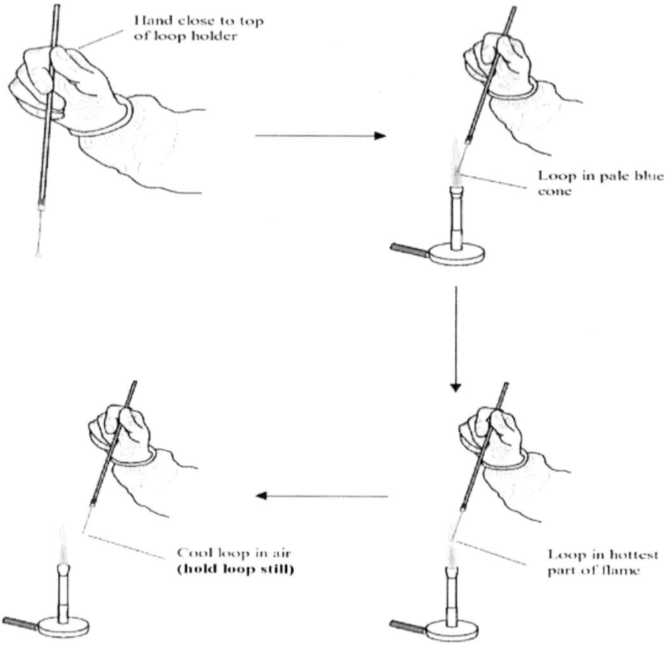

3. Using the loop, take a drop of the liquid culture medium (broth) provided and spread it carefully in a line across the surface of the agar as shown. With the same loop, a second, third and fourth line may be drawn parallel to the first. Close the lid of the petri dish immediately.
4. Sterilize the loop in the flame once again and allow it to cool.
5. Turn the petri dish so that the end of the previous lines can be the start of the next ones.
6. Take a sterilized and cooled loop and make 2 or 3 streaks as before. Close the lid of the petri-dish immediately.
7. Repeat step 4, 5 and 6 until there is no more space round the edge (4 or 5 times), then finish off with a single zigzag streak across the middle.

8. Seal and label the petri dish with the culture reference and your name and the date. Place it in an inverted position in the incubator at an appropriate temperature.

Questions

Q1. Has the technique caused the micro organisms in the culture to become separated?

Q2. Was the original culture viable?

Q3. Was the original culture a pure culture?

Q4. How would you obtain a pure culture from your plate?

Date: Signature of Instructor

Isolation of Bacteria in Pure Culture

1. Streak Plate Method

a) Observation of Streak Plate Method

After an appropriate time, examine the petri dish without opening it and look for individual colonies. Draw it.

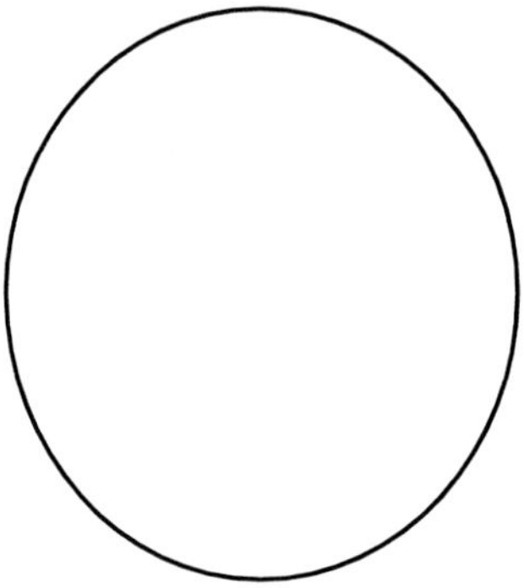

Result

Date: Signature of Instructor

2. Spot Method

Objective

1. To perform inoculation of bacteria by spot method.

Introduction

In this method, the bacterial inoculation is made in the form of a spot. This method is useful for procedures, such as phage typing and antimicrobial sensitivity testing.

Materials Required

Bacterial culture, inoculating loop, burner, nutrient agar plate (sterile), incubator.

Procedure

1. Sterilize loop and pick up a small amount of bacterial culture aseptically.
2. Raise the lid of the nutrient agar plate slightly and rub the inoculum at a spot on the surface of the medium.
3. Incubate the plate at 37^0C for 24-48 h.

Observation of Spot Method

Examine the plate and make drawing.

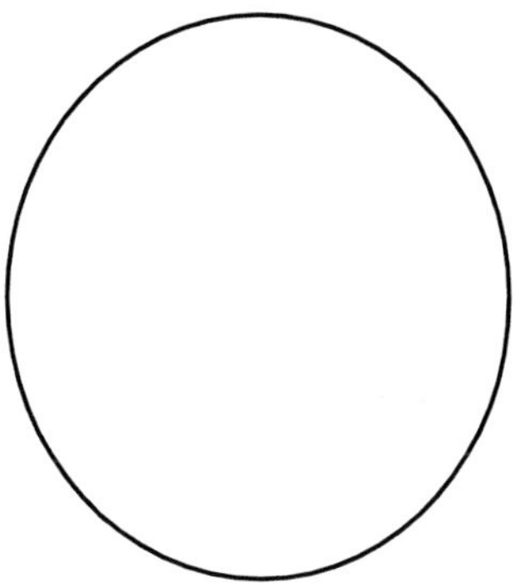

Result

Date: Signature of Instructor

3. Pour Plate Method

Objective

1. To perform bacterial inoculation by pour plate method.

Introduction

With the pour plate method, the bacteria are mixed with melted agar (at 45^{0}C) evenly distributed and separated throughout the liquid. The melted agar is then poured into an empty plate and allowed to solidify. After incubation, discrete bacterial colonies can then be found growing both on the agar and in the agar. This method is useful for obtaining pure bacterial culture from mixed inoculums and gives an estimate of the viable bacterial count in a suspension.

Materials Required

Bacterial broth culture, sterile nutrient broth tube (10 ml), sterile nutrient agar tube (15 ml), sterile petri dish, incubator, inoculating loop and water bath.

Procedure

1. Melt nutrient agar in a boiling water bath and cool to 46-48°C. This should not kill the bacteria when they are introduced to the liquid agar and will also reduce the amount of condensation that will collect on the lid of the Petri dish. Work quickly. The agar will solidify at 42°C.
2. Label the bottom of the sterile petri plate with the culture and your initials. Turn the plate, so the lid is facing up.
3. Aseptically add a loopful of broth culture in the nutrient broth tube and mix thoroughly.
4. Aseptically transfer a loopful of the diluted culture to the molten nutrient agar and rotate the tube rapidly for a few sec.
5. Pour the contents into a sterile petri dish and spread evenly; avoid creating air bubbles.
6. After the inoculated nutrient agar is solidified, incubate the plate at 37°C for 24-48 hours.

Questions

Q1. Mention any two disadvantages of this technique.

Observation of Pour Plate Method

Examine the plate and make drawing.

Result

Date: Signature of Instructor

4. Stroke Culture Method

Objective

1. To inoculate an agar slant by stroke culture method.

Introduction

The agar slants are inoculated using a sterile inoculating loop/ straight wire to streak the inoculum down the centre of the slant and then the inoculum is spreaded in a zigzag pattern. This is also known as 'stroke culture'.

Materials Required

Bacterial broth culture, inoculating loop, burner, sterile nutrient agar slant, incubator.

Procedure

1. Sterilize the loop and pick up a small amount of bacterial culture.
2. Insert the loop near the bottom of the slant and draw it gently upwards over the surface of the medium in a zigzag manner. Do not penetrate the agar.
3. Incubate the slant at 37°C for 24-48 h.

Observation of Stroke Culture Method

Result

Date: Signature of Instructor

5. Stab Method

Objective

1. To inoculate butt by stab method.

Introduction

A 4" long, thick sterile straight wire is used to inoculate a stab medium, for example motility indole urea (MIU) medium or gelatine medium. The medium is stabbed in the centre, taking care to withdraw the wire along the line of inoculums without making further stab lines.

Materials Required

Bacterial broth culture, sterile gelatine butt/agar butt, straight inoculation needle, burner, incubator.

Procedure

1. Sterilize inoculation needle and pick up a small amount of bacterial culture.
2. With aseptic precautions, remove the cotton plug from the agar tube and introduce the inoculation needle perpendicularly into the medium without touching the sides or bottom of the tube. Withdraw the needle through the same path without breaking the medium.
3. Incubate the tube at 37°C for 24-48 h.

Observation of Stab Method

Result

Date: Signature of Instructor

❑❑❑

Exercise 5

Cultivation of Aerobic and Anaerobic Bacteria

Objective

1. To study the oxygen requirements for aerobic cultivation of bacteria.

Introduction

Bacterial growth is dependent on the presence of oxygen, as different bacteria have different oxygen requirements depending on the types of enzymes they possess. The major classes of bacteria according to oxygen requirements are:

1. Obligate aerobic bacteria- compulsorily require oxygen for growth. e.g. *Nocardia, Mycobacterium tuberculosis, Pseudomonas aeruginosa.*
2. Obligate anaerobic bacteria- strictly requires absence of oxygen for growth. e.g. *Clostridium sp.*
3. Facultative bacteria- can grow in both presence/absence of bacteria. e.g. *Staphylococcus sp., E.coli, Listeria sp.*
4. Microaerophiles- require O_2 at below atmospheric concentrations, typically 2-10%. e.g. *Borrelia, Helicobacter pylori, Campylobacter.*
5. Aerotolerant- grow equally well in the presence and absence of oxygen. e.g. *Propionibacterium, Lactobacillus.*

Principle

Different types of bacteria on the basis of oxygen requirement can be identified by growing them in a liquid culture:

1. Obligate aerobic bacteria- They require atmospheric oxygen (20%) and use oxygen as the final electron acceptor in the electron

transport system. Thus, when grown in liquid culture the bacteria gather at the top of the test tube in order to absorb maximum amount of oxygen.

2. Obligate anaerobic bacteria : They cannot survive in the presence of any oxygen. Obligate anaerobes lack the enzymes necessary to breakdown the toxic by-products of oxygen. In these bacteria, the final electron acceptor in the electron transport system is a molecule other than oxygen. Thus, when grown in liquid culture the bacteria gather at the bottom to avoid oxygen.

3. Facultative bacteria : They are also able to live either in the presence or absence of oxygen, but they prefer oxygen, so they can carry out aerobic respiration with O_2 as final electron acceptor to maximize ATP yields. These organisms can use other electron acceptors if O_2 is not available, such as fumarate and nitrate. They can also utilize fermentative metabolism in the absence of oxygen. Thus, when grown in liquid media, the bacteria gather mostly at the top, since aerobic respiration is the most highly beneficial one, but as lack of oxygen does not affect them, they can be found all along the test tube.

4. Microaerophiles : They require oxygen at below atmospheric concentrations, typically 2-10%. They have a limited ability to neutralize toxic oxygen, so excess oxygen will kill the bacteria. However, microaerophiles do use oxygen as final acceptor in the electron transport system. Thus, when grown in liquid media, the bacteria gather at the upper part of the test tube but not at the top.

5. Aerotolerant : They grow equally well in the presence or absence of oxygen. They do possess enzymes necessary to neutralize toxic oxygen by-products, but they never use O_2 as a final electron acceptor. Thus, when grown in liquid media, the bacteria are not affected at all by oxygen and they are evenly spread along the test tube.

Materials Required

Brain Heart Infusion (BHI) deeps, bacterial culture, inoculating loop, burner, water bath and incubator.

Procedure

1. Melt the BHI agar tubes in a water bath.
2. While the BHI tube is still liquefied, inoculate the tube with bacterial culture.
3. Roll the tube between the palms of your hands to disperse the bacteria throughout the tube, taking care not to create bubbles.
4. Let the BHI tubes solidify.
5. Place the tube in incubator at 37°C for 48 hours.

Questions

Q1. A deep punctured wound will be attacked by what type of bacteria?

Q2. If a mixed culture of bacteria is inoculated in agar tube, which type of bacteria will grow at top, bottom and middle.

Observation of Aerobic Cultivation of Bacteria

Examine the BHI deep tubes for presence/absence of microbial growth and locate the growth in tubes below:

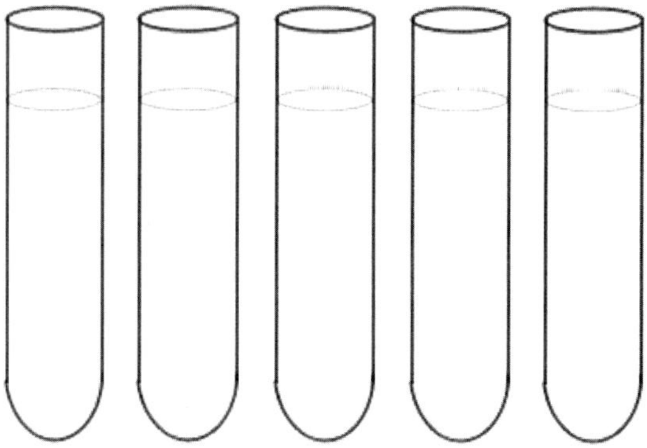

Result

Date: Signature of Instructor

Anaerobic Cultivation of Bacteria

Different methods are used for creating anaerobiosis for the growth of anaerobic bacteria in the absence of oxygen, e.g.

1. Candle jar
2. McIntosh & Filde's Anaerobic jar
3. Gas pak jar
4. Anaerobic media-such as Thioglycollate broth, Robertson cooked meat media.

I. Candle jar

A candle jar is a container in to which a lit candle is introduced before sealing the container's air tight lid. The candle's flame burns until extinguished by oxygen deprivation, which creates a carbon-dioxide rich, Oxygen poor atmosphere in the jar.

II. McIntosh Jar

It works on the principle of evacuation and replacement, where the air inside the chamber is evacuated and replaced with hydrogen or a mixture of gases. It consists of a glass or metal jar with a lid that can be tightly clamped with a screw to make it air tight. The lid has 2 taps, one acts as outlet that is connected to a vacuum pump and the other as inlet through which hydrogen gas is supplied. The lid also consists of two electrical terminals, which is connected on the underside to a small porcelain spool wrapped by a layer of palladinised asbestos. The inoculated culture plates are placed inside a metal jar and the lid clamped tight.

III.Gas Pak jar

It is a much simpler technique than the McIntosh and Filde's jar where one needs to pump gases in and out. There are commercially available, use and throw sachets containing a dry powder or pellets, which when mixed with water and kept in an appropriately sized air tight jar, produce an atmosphere free of elemental oxygen gas. The gas pak sachets consists of:

i) Sodium borohydrite-$NaBH_4$

ii) Sodium bicarbonate-$NaHCO_3$

iii) Citric acid-C_3H_5O $(COOH)_3$

iv) Cobalt chloride-$CoCl_2$ (catalyst)

These chemicals react with water to produce hydrogen and carbon dioxide. In an air tight gas jar the culture media , the gas pak sachet (opened and water added) and an indicator are placed. The jar is incubated at the desired temperature. A chemical indicator - Methylene blue is used to check whether anaerobiosis is created or not. On oxidation, in the presence of oxygen it is coloured deep blue, whereas becomes colourless, when oxygen is depleted and anaerobic conditions are achieved.

a) Thioglycollate Broth- It is a medium designed to test the aerotolerance of bacteria. Along with nutrients to support bacterial growth, it contains sodium thioglycollate, thioglycollic acid, L-cystine and methylene blue. The sodium thioglycollate, thioglycollic acid and L-cystine reduce the oxygen to water. Methylene blue is an indicator that is colourless in an anaerobic environment and blue in the presence of oxygen.

b) Robertson's cooked meat media- This medium was originally developed by Robertson for the cultivation of certain anaerobes. It supports the growth of many spore forming and non-spore forming strict anaerobes. It consists of beef heart, the muscle protein, which provide amino acids and other nutrients. Beef heart also contains glutathione, a reducing substance that permits the growth of obligate anaerobes. The sulphydryl groups, which impart reducing effect are more available in denatured protein and hence cooked meat is added in the medium. The addition of dextrose allows rapid and heavy growth of anaerobic bacteria in a short time and leads to more rapid identification of important anaerobes. Growth in this medium is indicated by turbidity or bubble formation. Blackening and disintegration of the meat particles indicate proteolysis.

Questions

Q1. Name any two anaerobic bacteria.

Q2. How much time does a candle take to extinguish in a candle jar?

Date: Signature of Instructor

Morphology and Cultural Characteristics

One of the major features of a bacterial strain is appearance of its growth in liquid and on solid media, known as 'cultural characteristics'. These growth characteristics are of taxonomic value and usually studied on the media, such as nutrient agar and nutrient broth. Observations are usually made after 24 hours of incubation under optimal conditions for growth, and subsequently at defined time intervals. Some of the main features are described below:

Surface colonies on agar plate

1. Size- In mm (pin point to large colonies of 5 mm or more in diameter); well-separated colonies must be measured and duration of growth should be stated.
2. Amount of growth- Scanty, moderate and abundant.
3. Shape/Form- Punctiform (Forms numerous very small 'pinpoint' colonies), circular, irregular, filamentous (long, irregular interwoven threads), spindle, rhizoid (irregular, branched)
4. Elevation- Sunken, flat, raised, convex, pulvinate, umbonate (convex with a central knob).
5. Margin/edge- Entire (smooth, no notches), undulate (wavy), Lobate (with alternate lobes and sinuses), lobed, filamentous (irregular, interwoven edges), rhizoid (root like).
6. Surface texture- Smooth (shining, glistening), rough (dull, granular), contoured (irregular, undulating), concentric/ringed (rings with common centre), wrinkled, papillate.
7. Optical characteristics- Opaque (not permitting light to pass through), translucent (some light passes through but not enough to permit visibility), opalescent (opal-like appearance, milky), transparent (light passes through completely), iridescent (exhibiting changing rainbow colours in reflected light).
8. Consistency- Butyrous (butter like), viscous (stingy, sticky), friable, rubbery, dry, brittle, powdery. This can be determined by touching a transfer needle to the colony.
9. Emulsifiability- Easy or difficult, form homogeneous or granular suspension in a loopful of normal saline solution.
10. Pigmentation- Present or absent. If present-colour of colonies (specific, fluorescent).

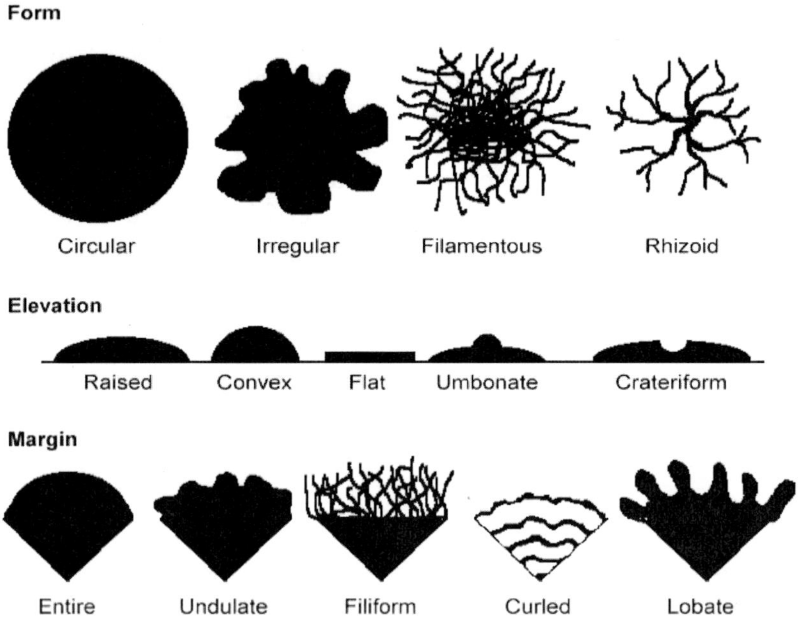

Diagram of colony morphology

Growth on agar slant

1. Amount/degree of growth- Sparse, moderate, abundant.
2. Form- Filiform (uniform growth along the line of inoculation), echinulate (growth along the line of inoculation with toothed or pointed margins), beaded (separate or semi confluent colonies along the line of streaking), effuse/spreading (growth extending much beyond the line of inoculation, i.e. several mm or more). Arborescent (branched, tree-like growth), rhizoid (growth with root-like margins).
3. Elevation- raised or diffused.
4. Edge
5. Surface texture
6. Optical characteristics
7. Consistency
8. Emulsifiability
9. Pigmentation

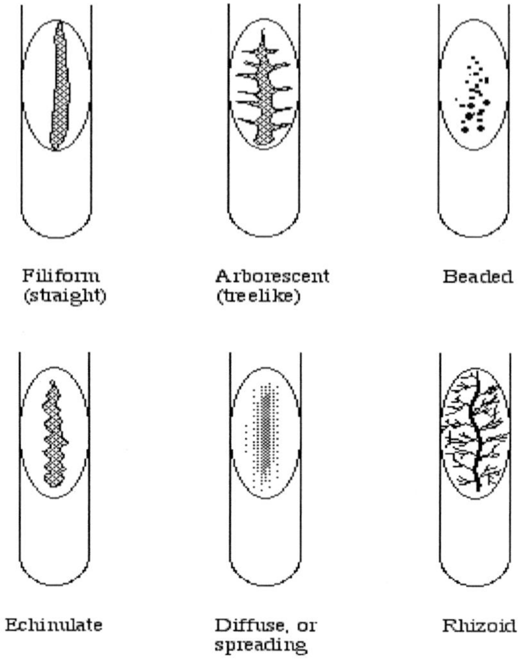

Diagram of growth in agar stab

Growth in agar stab

A stab culture is prepared by stabbing a solid medium, such as Nutrient gelatine, to almost the complete depth of the column with a charged straight wire. The following observations are made:

1. Amount of growth – scanty, moderate and abundant.
2. Form - filiform, beaded, papillate, arborescent.
3. Liquefaction (in case of gelatin stab) – crateriform (like a cup), napiform (like a turnip), saccate form (tubular), infundibuliform (like a funnel), stratiform (forming a layer), none (absent).
4. Surface growth – absent, present, pigmented.

Growth in broth culture

1. Amount of growth – scanty, moderate and abundant.
2. Surface growth – ring, pellicle, flocculent, membranous, absent.
3. Turbidity/Clouding – present/ absent.

4. Sediment/Deposit – present (compact, flocculent, granular, flaky, viscid), absent.
5. Odour – present, absent.
6. Pigmentation – present, absent.
7. Gas – present, absent.

Date: Signature of Instructor

Biochemical Characteristics

(A) Catalase Test

Objective

1. To perform catalase test.

Principle

Catalase is the name of an enzyme found in most bacteria, which initiates the breakdown of hydrogen peroxide (H_2O_2) into water (H_2O) and free oxygen (O_2). Most bacteria are catalase-positive; however, certain genera that don't carry out aerobic respiration, such as Streptococcus, Lactobacillus, and Clostridium, are catalase-negative.

Materials Required

Bacterial Cultures, 3% hydrogen peroxide.

Procedure

1. Place a drop of 3% hydrogen peroxide on a clean slide.
2. Using a sterile loop, pick a small amount of one of your test bacteria from your plate and emulsify in the drop of H_2O_2.
3. Look carefully to see if bubbles form, indicating the presence of the enzyme catalase.

Interpretation

If the organism has catalase activity, foaming or effervescence (bubbles) will appear within 10-30 seconds.

Date: Signature of Instructor

Oxidase Test

Objective

1. To perform oxidase test.

Principle

A positive oxidase reaction reflects the ability of a micro organism to oxidize certain aromatic amines, such as teratethyl-phenylenediamine (TPD), producing coloured end products. This is due to the activity of cytochrome oxidase in the presence of atmospheric oxygen. One use of the test is for the preliminary identification of Neisseria and Moraxella species, which are both oxidase positive gram-negative diplococcic. Members of Enterobacteriaceae are oxidase negative.

Materials Required

Bacterial Cultures, 1% aqueous solution tetramethyl-p-phenylenediamine, wooden stick.

Procedure

1. Obtain 2 oxidase test strips or discs.
2. Using a sterile PLASTIC loop, pick a small amount of bacterial culture from your plate and smear it on the test area of the disc.
3. Colour change should occur rapidly—yellow/buff is a negative result, purple is a positive result.

Result

Date: Signature of Instructor

Sugar Fermentation Test

Objective

1. To perform sugar fermentation test.

Principle

Certain bacteria attack a characteristic range of carbohydrates producing acidity, detected by an indicator, and sometimes gas, detected by a submerged, inverted Durham tube.

Constituents of fermentation test media

1. A suitable nutrient medium, such as peptone water, as a base to allow the growth of the organism under test, free from substances that might yield acid products. The nature of this medium depends on the nutritional requirements of the organism. Peptone water, serum peptone water and serum agar are commonly used.
2. The carbohydrates or related compound under test. A large variety is used and they are often referred to loosely as 'sugars'.
3. A suitable indicator that will change colour as a result of the formation of acids during the fermentation. Some common examples are Andrade's indicator (used at a final concentration of 0.005%), bromocresol purple (used at a final concentration of 0.005%), phenol red (used at a final concentration of 0.01%), and bromothymol blue (used at a final concentration of 0.0025%). Bromothymol blue is used in preference to Andrade's indicator because it does not fade quickly.
4. A small inverted tube, known as Durham tube completely filled with liquid and containing no air bubbles is usually included in each culture tube or bottle to detect gas.

Materials Required

Peptone water culture of *E.coli* and *S.*Typhimurium, sterile peptone water fermentation test media with different sugars, Durham tube, and sterile Pasteur pipette.

Composition of Peptone water sugar

Peptone	10.0 g
Sodium chloride	5.0 g
Bromothymol blue*, 2g/1 (0.2% w/v)	12.5 ml
Distilled water	1000.0 ml

*Prepared by dissolving 0.1 of bromothymol blue in 2.5ml of N/10 sodium hydroxide. Add 47.5ml of sterile distilled water and mix well. Store in the dark.

1. Dissolve the peptone and salt in the water. Adjust the pH to 7.2-7.3. Add the indicator solution.
2. Dispense in 100 ml amounts in screw-cap bottles and sterilize by autoclaving (with caps loosened) at 121^{0}C for 15 min. When cool, tighten the bottle caps.

5% peptone water sugar

Sterile peptone water with indicator	100.0 ml
Sterile 10% w/v sugar solution*	5.0 ml

*Prepared by dissolving 2.5 g of the sugar in 100 ml of distilled water and sterilised by filtration or steaming for 30 minutes. Alternatively, buy the ampoules containing 5 ml of sterile 10% sugar solution or discs impregnated with sugar from commercial suppliers.

1. Add aseptically the sterile sugar solution to the sterile peptone water-containing indicator, and mix well.
2. Dispense aseptically in 4 ml amounts in sterile Bijou bottles containing an inverted Durham tube (sterilized with the bottle). The pH of medium should be near pH 7.6, which will give the medium a blue colour; bromothymol blue indicator becomes yellow at pH 6.0.

Procedure

1. Label sugar tubes properly in a rack (3 each).
2. With the help of a sterile Pasteur pipette, inoculate one tube of each sugar with two drops of *E. coli* culture.

3. Repeat step 2 with culture of S. Typhimurium. Keep third tube of each sugar as uninoculated control.
4. Incubate the tubes at 37⁰C for at least 48 h or longer, if required.

Interpretation

Yellow	Acid produced
Blue	Acid not produced (no colour change)

Gas is detected as the air bubble in the inverted Durham tube.

Result

Date: Signature of Instructor

Methyl Red Test

Objective

1. To perform methyl red test.

Principle

This test is employed to detect production of sufficient acids during fermentation of glucose resulting in pH below 4.5 and its sustained maintenance during period of incubation. Consequently upon addition of methyl red indicator (pH range: 4.0-6.2) red colour appears in the reaction tube. The test is preformed to differentiate members of the family Enterobacteriaceae. As some organisms may further metabolise the acids to various neutral products, the duration of incubation period is very important.

Materials Required

Cultures of *E. coli* and *Klebsiella*, glucose phosphate peptone water tubes, methyl red indicator.

Glucose Phosphate water

Peptone	0.5 g
Glucose (dextrose)	0.5 g
Di-potassium hydrogen phosphate (K_2HPO_4)	0.5 g
Distilled water	100.0 ml

1. Dissolve the peptone and phosphate salt in the water by steaming. When cooled, filter and adjust the pH to 7.5.
2. Add the glucose and mix well.
3. Dispense the medium in 1.5 ml amounts in small screw-cap tubes or bottles.
4. Sterilise by autoclaving (with caps loosened) at 121°C for 10 min. When cool, tighten the container tops.

Methyl red indicator

Methyl red	0.1 g
Ethanol	300.0 ml
Distilled water	200.0 ml

Procedure

1. Inoculate one tube of phosphate peptone water with *E.coli* culture and the other with *Klebsiella pneumoniae*. Keep third tube as control.
2. Incubate all tubes at 37^{0}C for 48 h.
3. Add 5 drops of methyl red indicator in each culture tube and also in one uninoculated control tube for comparing the colour.

Interpretation

Red	Positive
Yellow	Negative
Orange	Doubtful

Result

Date: Signature of Instructor

Voges – Proskauer (Acetoin) Test

Objective

1. To differentiate enterobacteria.

Principle

Certain bacteria ferment carbohydrates to produce acetyl methyl carbinol (CH_3.CHOH.CO.CH_3) or its reduction product 2,3 butylene glycol (CH_3.CHOH.CO.CH_3) from pyruvic acid in the medium, which can be detected by colorimetric methods. Following addition of alkali and then vigorous shaking of the tube, acetyl methyl carbinol or 2, 3 butylene glycol is oxidised to diacetyl. Diacetyl reacts with the guanidine or arginine present in the medium (peptone) and produces a pink red colour.

The test is usually done in conjunction with the methyl red test since the production of acetyl methyl carbinol or butylenes glycol usually result in insufficient acid accumulation during fermentation to give a methyl red positive reaction. An organism of the Enterobacteriaceae family group is usually either MR positive or VP negative or vice-versa.

Method 1

Materials Required

Cultures of *E.coli* and *Kleb. pneumoniae*, glucose phosphate water, 5% alcoholic solution of α-naphthol and 40% aqueous of potassium hydroxide.

Procedure

1. Inoculate one tube of glucose phosphate peptone water with *E.coli* culture and the other with *Kleb.pneumoniae*.
2. Incubate the inoculated tubes at 37°C for 48 to 72 h.
3. Add 0.6 ml of α-naphthol and 0.2 ml of potassium hydroxide solution to ml of each culture. Shake thoroughly, slope the tube and examine after 15 min and 1 h.

Interpretation

Pink - red	Positive test (acetoin produced)
No - pink - red colour	Negative test (No acetoin produced)

Result

Date: Signature of Instructor

Citrate Utilization Test

Objective

1. To differentiate enterobacteria from other bacteria.

Principle

The test organism is cultured in a medium containing sodium citrate, ammonium salt and bromothymol blue indicator. The organism use citrate (the only source of carbon) and ammonia (the only source of nitrogen). The citrate utilisation is followed by alkaline reaction (change of the colour from light green to blue) and growth in the medium is indicated by appearance of turbidity.

Materials Required

Cultures of *Kleb. pneumoniae* and *E. coli,* citrate medium.

Simmon's method

Composition

Koser's medium	1.0 l
Agar	20.0 g
Bromothymol blue 0.2% solution	40.0 ml

Dispense autoclave at 121^{0}C for 15 min and allow setting as slope.

Procedure

Inoculate as a single streak lightly over the surface of slant and incubate at 37^{0}C. Examine daily for up to 7 days for growth and colour change. Confirm positive result by sub culturing to the same medium.

Interpretation

Blue colour and streak of growth	Positive test
Original green colour and no growth	Negative test

Result

Date: Signature of Instructor

Oxidation – Fermentation (O/F) Test

(Hugh and Leifson's method)

Objective

1. To determine the oxidative or fermentative metabolism of a carbohydrate by the bacterium.

Introduction

The medium is semi-solid and usually contains glucose as the test sugar and bromothymol blue as the pH indicator. This test is used to differentiate those organisms that oxidise carbohydrates (aerobic utilisations), such as *Pseudomonas aeruginosa,* from those organisms that ferment carbohydrates (anaerobic utilisation), such as members of the Enterobacteriaceae.

Principle

The test organisms is inoculated into two tubes of a tryptone or peptone agar medium containing glucose (or other carbohydrate) and the indicator bromothymol blue. The inoculated medium in one tube is sealed with a layer of liquid paraffin to exclude oxygen.

Fermentative organisms utilise carbohydrate in both the open and sealed tubes as shown by a change in colour of the medium from green to yellow. Oxidative organism, however, are able to use the carbohydrate only in the open tube. There is no carbohydrate utilization in the sealed tube (medium remains green).

Although most genera of aerobics are either carbohydrate oxidisers or fermenter, the productions of acid may be slow and, therefore cultures are usually incubated for 7-14 days.

Some bacteria are unreactive in the conventional O-F medium, either because they are unable to grow in the medium basal medium or because they cannot attack glucose.

Materials Required

Cultures of *E.coli* and *Pseudomonas aeruginosa,* O-F medium, sterile liquid paraffin (paraffin oil), nichrome straight wire.

Composition (O-F Medium)

Tryptone or peptone	2.0 g
Sodium chloride	5.0 g
Di-Potassium hydrogen phosphate anhydrous (K_2HPO_4)	0.3 g
Agar	2.5 g
Bromothymol blue, 10g/l (1% w/v)	3.0 ml
Distilled water	1.0 l

*Prepared by dissolving 0.5 g in 50 ml of distilled water

1. Mix the dry ingredients in the water and heat to 100°C to dissolve (Place the flask in a container of boiling water). Adjust the pH to 7.1.
2. Allow to cool to 50-55°C and then add 3 ml of the bromothymol blue indicator. Mix well.
3. Dispense in 50 ml amounts in screw-cap containers. Sterilise by autoclaving (with caps loosened) at 121°C for 15 minutes.
4. Cool to 50-55°C and then add aseptically 5ml of a sterile 10% w/v glucose (dextrose) solution. Mix well.
5. Dispense aseptically in 9 ml amounts in sterile screw-cap tubes or bottles.

Procedure

1. Using a sterile straight wire, inoculate the test organism to the bottom of two tubes of sterile O-F medium. Use heavy inoculums. Before inoculation heat the tubes in a beaker of boiling water bath to drive off any dissolved oxygen.
2. Cover the inoculated wire; inoculate the test organism to the tubes with a 10 mm deep layer of sterile paraffin oil to seal it from air.
3. Incubate the tubes at 35-37°C for upto 14 days. Examine daily for carbohydrates utilizations as shown by acid production.

Interpretation

Open tube	**Sealed tube**	**Interpretation**	**Example**
Yellow	Green	Oxidative organism	*Pseudomonas* spp.
Yellow	Yellow	Fermentative organism	*E.coli*
Green or blue	Green	No utilization of carbohydrates	*Bordetella* spp.

Result

Date: Signature of Instructor

Gelatine Liquefaction

Objective

1. To perform the gelatin liquefaction test.

Principle

Gelatin is a protein, which is liquefied by gelatinase enzyme produced by some bacteria. Liquefied gelatine cannot from a gel. The criterion of gelatine liquefaction helps in the identification of certain species of bacteria.

Materials Required

Cultures of *Proteus* spp. and *E.coli*, gelatine tubes, nichrome straight wires.

Composition

Gelatine medium

Gelatine	120.0 g
Distilled water	1000.0 ml

1. Dissolve gelatine in 100 ml of distilled water by heating.
2. Dispense in 7 ml amount in test tubes (15 x 125 mm).
3. Sterilise by autoclaving at 115^{0}C for 20 min.

Nutrient Gelatin

Meat extract	3.0 g
Peptone	5.0 g
Gelatine	120.0 g
Water	1000.0 ml

1. Add the gelatine to the water and allow standing for 15-30 min.
2. Heat to dissolve the gelatine, do not overheat.
3. Add and dissolve the other ingredients.
4. Adjust to pH 7.0 and dispense in test tubes.
5. Sterilise by autoclaving at 115^{0}C for 20 min.

Procedure

1. Inoculate one gelatine tube with *Proteus* spp and the other tube with *E.coli* by stabbing using a straight wire. The third tube will act as uninoculated control.
2. Incubate all three tubes at 37⁰C for upto 14 days; incubation at 20⁰C for longer period is preferred, if the organisms can grow at this temperature.
3. After every 2-3 days place all gelatine tubes in a refrigerator for 2 h or till the medium of the control tube solidifies. Compare the medium of the inoculated tubes with that of control tube.

Interpretation

Liquefied gelatine does not solidify on refrigeration.

Result

Date: Signature of Instructor

Digestion of Milk (Casein Hydrolysis)

Objective

1. To perform the casein hydrolysis test.

Principle

Casein is an exoenzyme that is produced by some bacteria in order to degrade casein. Casein is a large protein that is responsible for the white colour of milk. This test is conducted on milk agar which is a complex media containing casein, peptone and beef extract. If an organism can produce casein, then there will be a zone of clearing around the bacterial growth.

Materials Required

Cultures of *Bacillus subtilis* and *Escherichia coli*, casein milk agar.

Composition

Nutrient agar, sterile	87.5 ml
Skimmed milk	12.5 ml
(sterilised at 115^{0}C for 10 min)	

Melt the agar, cool to 50^{0}C, add the milk and pour plates.

Procedure

Divide the Skim Milk agar plate in half and inoculate one half with *Bacillus subtilis* and the other half with *Escherichia coli*. Incubate at 37^{0}C for 10-14 days.

Interpretation

Zone of clearing around colonies	Positive test
No clearing	Negative test

Observation

Result

Date: Signature of Instructor

Hydrogen Sulphide Production (Keigler's Test)

Objective

1. To detect the liberation of H_2S gas by bacteria.

Introduction

Hydrogen sulphide is produced by bacterial anaerobic degradation of the two sulphur containing amino acids, cysteine and methionine. It is released as a by-product when carbon and nitrogen atoms in the amino acids are consumed as nutrients by the cells. Under anaerobic conditions, the sulphydryl (-SH) group on cysteine is reduced by cysteine desulphurase.

Principle

Production of hydrogen sulphide by the micro organisms is tested in the medium containing sulphur compounds like cystine, methionine and glutathione. Bacteria may be grown in ordinary broth, peptone water or in any other medium containing sulphur compounds. Hydrogen sulphide produce by the breakdown of sulphur compounds can be detected by the incorporation of a heavy metal salt (e.g., lead iron, etc.) into the medium. Hydrogen sulphide reacts with the metal to from black metal sulphides. The production of H_2S is usually detected by hanging a lead acetate filter paper strip in the culture tube. Hydrogen sulphide liberated from the medium will act on the lead acetate filter paper changing its white colour to black. The reaction is shown below:

$$(CH_3COO)_2Pb + H_2S \rightarrow PbS + 2CH_3COOH$$

Lead acetate Lead sulphide Acetic acid

For H_2S production excessive aeration in the culture should be avoided.

Materials Required

Cultures of *E. coli* and *Proteus vulgaris*, nutrient broth or peptone water tubes, sterile filter paper strips saturated with lead acetate.

Preparation of strips

1. Cut 5–10 mm (wide) x 50–60 mm (long) strips of filter paper.
2. Soak the strips in lead acetate (tri-hydrate salt) hot saturated aqueous solution (10 g lead acetate in 100 ml hot water).
3. Dry at 50 to 60^{0}C and store in airtight containers.

Procedure

Inoculate one tube with *E. coli* another tube with *Proteus vulgaris*. Insert a strip of lead acetate filter paper in between the side of the tube and cotton plug so that it hangs freely into the tube up to the height of about an inch from the top of the medium. Incubate at 37^{0}C for 10-14 days.

Interpretation

Hydrogen sulphide production will turn the paper brown or black by converting lead acetate to lead sulphide.

Result

Date: Signature of Instructor

Indole Test

Objective

1. To perform indole test.

Principle

Bacteria utilise various acids as their food. Some bacteria use the enzyme tryptophanase to convert the amino acid tryptophan into molecules of indole, pyruvic acid and ammonia. Since only a few bacteria contain tryptophanase, the formation of indole from a tryptophan substrate can be another useful diagnostic tool for the identification of an organism. Indole production is a key test for the identification of *Escherichia coli*.

Testing for indole production is important in the identification of enterobacteria. Four metabolic tests, viz. Indole production, methyl red test, Voges – Proskauer reaction and citrate utilization, collectively known as IMViC tests, are used to differentiate members of Enterobacteriaceae family.

Result

Date: Signature of Instructor

Kovac's method

Materials Required

Peptone water tubes, cultures of *E.coli* and *Kleb.pneumoniae*, Kovac's reagent.

Composition

p-dimethyl amino benzaldehyde	0.5 g
Amyl or isoamyl alcohol	75.0 ml
Conc. HCI	25.0 ml

Dissolve the aldehyde in the alcohol and slowly add the acid. Store in brown bottle at 4^0C.

Procedure

1. Inoculate one peptone water tube with *E.coli* and another with *Kleb. pneumoniae*.
2. Incubate at 37^0C for 48 h.
3. Add 0.5ml Kovac's reagent and shake gently.

Interpretation

A red colour in the alcohol layer indicates a positive reaction.

Result

Date: Signature of Instructor

Urease Test

Objective

1. To perform urease test.

Principle

Some bacteria produce the enzyme urease, which breakdown the urea (by hydrolysis) present in the medium to give ammonia and carbon dioxide. With the release of ammonia, the medium because alkaline due to which the colour of the indicator (phenol red) added in the medium change from yellow to pink or red. Urease test is useful for differentiating enterobacteria; Proteus stains are urease positive while salmonellae and shigellae do not produce this enzyme.

$$NH_2\ CONH_2 \rightarrow 2NH_3 + CO_2$$

Urea +H_2O Ammonia

Materials Required

Culture of Proteus and Salmonella and urea agar.

Composition

Peptone	1.0 g
Sodium chloride	5.0 g
Potassium monohydrogen (or dihydrogen) phosphate	2.0 g
Agar	20.0 g
Distilled water	1.0 l

Dissolve the ingredients by heating; adjust the pH to 6.8 and autoclave at 121⁰C for 15 min. and cool to 50⁰C.

Glucose	1.0 g
Phenol red (0.2% solution)	6.0 ml
Add to the molten base, steam for 1h, and cool to 50⁰C.	
Urea, 20% soln. (sterilised by filtration)	100.0 ml

Mix well and prepare slants.

Procedure

1. Inoculate one slant with Proteus and other with Salmonella.
2. Incubate at 37^{0}C for 24 to 48h.

Interpretation: A change in colour of the medium to pink or red indicates a positive reaction.

Result

Date: Signature of Instructor

❑❑❑

Exercise **6**

Simple Staining

Objective

1. To recognize the three basic shapes of bacterial cells.

Introduction

Bacterial specimens are often stained prior to microscopy studies, which allow better visualization of specimens using microscopy. Simply speaking, a stain is a substance that adheres to a cell, giving the cell colour. Different stains have different affinities for different organisms, or different parts of organisms. They may be used to differentiate different types of organisms or to view specific parts of organisms.

There are several types of stains which are commonly used in microbiology. The first is a Simple stain, which uses only one reagent which provides contrast between the background and the heat fixed bacterium itself. The bacterium takes up stain and becomes coloured, while the background remains unstained. Simple stains, such as methylene blue, crystal violet, carbol fuchsin, etc. are typically used on bacterial smears which have been heat fixed and thus, contain non-living microbes.

Principle

In order to observe most bacterial cells using bright field microscopy the cells must be dark enough to see, that is they must have contrast to the light. To create contrast a simple stain can be used. Simple stains use basic dyes which are positively charged. These positive dyes interact with the slightly negatively charged bacterial cell wall, thus lending the colour of the dye to the cell wall.

Materials Required

Microscope, slides, inoculating loop, broth culture of bacteria, stain, etc.

Procedure

1. Clean and dry microscope slides thoroughly.
2. Flame the inoculating loop.
3. Transfer a loop full of sterile broth to the slide surface.
4. Remove the test tube cap with the fingers of the hand holding the loop.
5. Flame the tube mouth.
6. With the help of an inoculating loop pick up a pin head size sample of the bacterial growth.
7. Reflame the tube mouth, replace the cap, and put the tube back in the holder.
8. Disperse the bacteria on the loop in the drop of broth on the slide and spread the drop over an area, so as to obtain a thin smear.
9. Reflame the inoculating loop to redness including the entire length that entered the tube.
10. Allow the smear to dry thoroughly.
11. Heats fix the smear cautiously by passing the underside of the slide through the burner flame two or three times. Test the temperature of the slide after each pass against the back of the hand. Heat fixation of bacterial smear accomplishes three things:
    i) It kills the organisms.
    ii) It causes the organisms to adhere to the slide and
    iii) It alters the organisms so that they more readily acquire the stain. Overheating will distort the cells.
12. Stain the smear by flooding it with on of the staining solutions an allowing it to remain covered with the stain for the time designated below:

    Methylene blue - 1 minute

    Crystal violet - 30 seconds

    Carbol fuchsin - 20 seconds

13. At the end of the designated time, rinse off the excess stain with gently running tap water. Rinse thoroughly.
14. Wipe the back of the slide and blot dry the stained surface.
15. Place the stained smear on the microscope stage smear side up and focus the smear using the 10X objective.
16. Choose an area of the smear in which the bacterial cells are well spread in a monolayer.
17. Center the area to be studied, apply cedar wood oil directly to the smear, and focus the smear under oil with the 100X objective.

Observation of Simple Staining

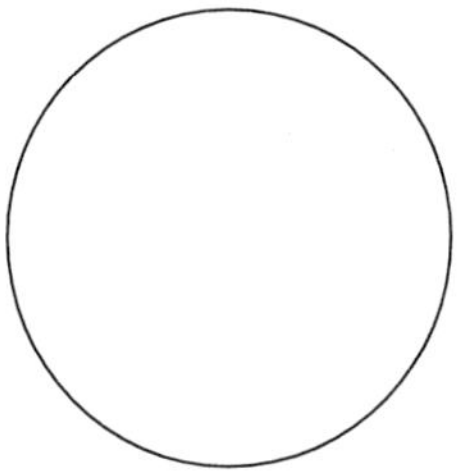

Result

Date: Signature of Instructor

Exercise 7

Negative Staining

Objective

1. To determine morphology, arrangement and size of bacteria, that may be affected by heat fixing by negative staining technique.

Introduction

Negative staining is a technique in which the background is stained, leaving the actual specimen, untouched, and thus visible. It is typically performed using a black ink fluid, such as Nigrosin/ India ink. This technique is mainly used to stain cells that are too delicate to be heat fixed. The advantages of the negative stain includes the use of only one stain and the absence of heat fixation of the sample.

Principle

The negative stain uses the dye nigrosin, which is an acidic dye. By giving up a proton (as an acid) the chromophore of the dye becomes negatively charged. Because the cell wall is also negatively charged only the background around the cells will become stained, leaving the cells unstained.

Materials Required

Microscope slides, nigrosin dye, bacterial culture, inoculating loop, dropper and microscope.

Procedure

1. Place a small drop of nigrosin stain at the end of a clean slide.
2. Using aseptic technique, mix a drop of broth culture (use a different one than in step 1) into the drop of nigrosin. Avoid spreading the drop or allowing it to dry out.

3. Hold the edge of another slide at an angle to the first slide and spread the drop out along the first slide so that a gradient of dye forms.
4. Let the dye smear air dry, but do NOT heat fix. This can distort the cells.
5. Observe your smear under the microscope and record your observations.

Interpretation

Transparent bacterial cells are visible on dark background.

Observation of Negative Staining

Observe your slide in the microscope under oil immersion and draw a few representative organisms below (use colour pencils):

Result

Questions

Q1. Could any dye be used in place of nigrosin in negative staining?

Q2. Why is the size more accurate in a negative stain than a simple stain?

Date: Signature of Instructor

Exercise 8

Differential Staining Procedures of Bacteria

A) Gram's Staining

Objective

1. To differentiate between the two major categories of bacteria: Gram positive and Gram negative.

Introduction

Gram staining is a method of differentiating bacteria according to their gram character (Gram positive or gram negative). It is one of the initial steps carried out in microbiological laboratories for the identification of etiological agent and hence, is one of the most important staining techniques in microbiology. This staining method is named after its inventor Hans Christian Gram.

Principle

Gram staining depends on the structure and composition of the cell wall of bacteria. Gram positive bacteria have thicker peptidoglycan layer than gram negative bacteria. First, primary stain, crystal violet stains all the cells purple. Addition of iodine (mordant) forms crystal violet iodine complex within the cell wall. The complex formed is larger than crystal violet, so it cannot be easily washed out from the intact peptidoglycan layer. Application of alcohol (decolourizer) decolourizes the stain. Since gram negative organism have thin peptidoglycan layer and have additional lipopolysaccharide layer which gets dissolved due to the additional alcohol, so gram negative organism fails to retain the complex and gets decolourized. On the other hand gram positive continues to retain the complex and remain purple. To observe the decolourized cells secondary stains like safranin is added which stains the gram negative organisms pink.

Materials Required

Primary stain- Crystal violet

Mordant – Gram's iodine

Decolourizer- 95% ethanol

Counter stain- Safranin

Glass slide, immersion oil, blotting paper, microscope, burner, water.

Procedure

1. Prepare a bacterial smear on a microscope glass slide.
2. Keep the slide over a staining rack and flood the smear with crystal violet and allow it to react for 1-2 minutes.
3. Wash the smear with running tap water.
4. Flood the smear with gram's iodine and allow to react for 1 minute.
5. Wash the smear with running tap water.
6. Decolourize the smear using 95% ethanol for 10-20 seconds.
7. Wash the smear with running tap water.
8. Counter stain with safranin for 30-60 seconds.
9. Wash the smear with running tap water.
10. Blot dry and focus the smear under low power, high dry and then oil immersion.

Precautions

1. Use clean glass slides.
2. Do not overheat.
3. Avoid excessive rinsing.
4. Make thin smears.
5. Be sure your cultures are young, preferably less than 24 hours old. Older cultures tend to lose the ability to retain stains.

Questions

Q1. What are the conditions when gram positive bacteria can appear gram negative?

Q2. If the iodine steps were omitted in the gram staining procedure, what colour would you expect gram positive and gram negative bacteria to stain?

Q3. Complete the following table:

S.No.	Stain/reagent	Colour of gram +ve bacteria	Colour of gram -ve bacteria
1.	Gram's Stain		
2.	Gram's Iodine		
3.	Decolourizer		
4.	Safranin		

Q.4. Which part of the bacteria actually gets stained?

Observation of Gram's staining

Observe your smear in the microscope under oil immersion and draw a few representative organisms from the smear below (use colour pencils):

Result

Date: Signature of Instructor

Exercise 9

Acid Fast Staining

Objective

1. To stain acid-fast bacilli by modified Ziehl-Nelson method.

Introduction

Acid fastness is a physical property of certain bacteria, specifically their resistance to decolourization by acids during staining procedures. Acid fast organisms, such as *Mycobacterium tuberculosis* and *Mycobacterium bovis* are difficult to characterize using standard microbiological techniques. Though they can be stained using concentrated dyes, particularly when the staining process is combined with heat. Acid-fast bacteria have a waxy substance called mycolic acid in their cell walls, which comprises upto 60% of the cell wall components. Once stained, these organisms resist the dilute acid and /or ethanol based decolourization procedures common in many staining protocols, hence the name acid fast.

Principle

The waxy mycolic acid containing cell wall of mycobacteria are relatively impermeable to ordinary staining techniques. They can be stained by aniline dyes using drastic measures, such as application of heat and phenol. Heat softens the wax in the cell wall and allows to stain (basic fuchsin) to enter. The fuchsin dye is more soluble in phenol than in water or alcohol. Phenol in turn is more soluble in lipids or waxes, thus the dye-phenol mixture enters the cell. Once stained, it resists decolourization by weak mineral acid (20% H_2SO_4). This is due to the fact that phenol–dye mixture is more soluble in waxes of the mycobacteria than the acid or alcohol. This way phenol acts as a mordant. While the mycobacteria retain the primary stain (pink), the background material gets decolourized and takes up the counterstain (methylene blue).

Materials Required

Primary stain- strong carbol fuchsin (consist of basic fuchsin and carbolic acid/phenol)

Decolourizer- 20% sulfuric acid (H_2SO_4) or acid alcohol.

Counter stain-Loeffler's methylene blue or malachite green

Glass slides, culture of acid fast bacteria or infected tissue sample, forcep, burner, microscope.

Procedure

1. Prepare a smear on a slide.
2. Air dry the smear and then heat fix it.
3. Flood the slide with carbol fuchsin.
4. Hold a flame beneath the slide until steam appears but do not allow it to boil.
5. Allow hot slide to stand for 3 to 5 minutes, rinse with tap water.
6. Flood the slide with acid alcohol.
7. Allow it to stand for 1 minute, rinse with tap water.
8. Flood the slide with counter stain Loffler's methylene blue solution for 1-2 minutes.
9. Wash the slide and dry.
10. Focus the slide and see under oil immersion.

Observation of Acid Fast Staining:

Observe your smear in the microscope under oil immersion and draw a few representative organisms from the smear below (use colour pencils);

Questions

Q1. What property of the cell is responsible for the acid-fast reaction?

Q2. Complete the following table:

S.No.	Stain/reagent	Colour of acid fast bacteria	Colour of non-acid fast bacteria
1.	Carbol Fuchsin		
2.	Decolourizer		
3.	Methylene Blue		

Q3. What is acid alcohol decolourizer?

Result

Date: Signature of Instructor

❑❑❑

Exercise **10**

Special Staining

A) Metachromatic Granules Staining

Objective

1. To stain metachromatic granules.

Introduction

Metachromatic granules are inclusion bodies in some bacterial cells that alter the colour of particular stains (metachromasia). For e.g. In Corynebacterium, the metachromatic granules are composed of polyphosphates and act as energy storage sites. They are also known as Volutin granules. Albert's staining technique is a type of special staining which is used to stain metachromatic granules.

Principle

Albert stain is used to demonstrate special structures such as metachromatic granules in bacteria. Metachromatic granules are commonly found in *Corynebacterium* species. Two solutions are used in Albert's staining–Albert I and II solutions. If the smear contain *Corynebacterium,* a green coloured rod shaped bacteria that are arranged at angle to each other, showing letter "L","V" are seen and it is attached with dark greenish blue metachromatic granules.

Materials Required

Corynebacterium culture, slide, Albert's I solution, Albert's II solution, staining rack, blotting paper, immersion oil, normal saline, burner, microscope, inoculating loop.

Composition of Albert I solution

Toluidine blue	0.15 g
Malachite green	0.20 g
Glacial acetic acid	1.00 ml
Alcohol (95%)	2.00 ml
Distilled water	100.00 ml

Composition of Albert II solution

Iodine	2.0 g
Potassium iodide	3.0 g
Distilled water	300.0 ml.

Procedure

1. Prepare a thin smear of the bacterial culture on a clean glass slide in normal saline solution, dry in air and fix the dried smear using alcohol.
2. Cover the smear with Albert stain I. Let it stand for two minutes.
3. Wash off the stain with clean water.
4. Cover the smear with Albert stain II. Let it stand for two minutes. Wash with water.
5. Wipe the back of the slide clean, and place in a draining rack for the smear to air-dry.
6. Examine the smear microscopically, first with the 40x objectives to check the staining and to see the distribution of material and then with the oil immersion lens to look for bacteria containing metachromatic granules.

Interpretation

The metachromatic granules will stain greenish blue and cells take green stain.

Special Staining

a) Observation of Metachromatic Granule's Staining

Observe your smear in the microscope under oil immersion and draw a few representative organisms from the smear below (use colour pencils):

Questions

Q1. Name the different ways to demonstrate metachromatic granules.

Q2. Why are the bacilli arranged at angles to each other?

Result

Date: Signature of Instructor

B) Capsular Staining

Objective

1. To reveal the presence of the bacterial capsule.

Introduction

The capsule stain is a type of differential stain which selectively stains bacterial capsules. A capsule is a substance that is synthesized in the cytoplasm and secreted to the outside of the cell where it surrounds the bacterium. Capsules can be polysaccharide, polypeptide, or glycoprotein. Capsules are associated with virulence in several microorganisms, including *Streptococcus pneumoniae* and *Neisseria meningitidis*, because capsules provide a mechanism for these pathogens to evade the host immune system. Because of their structure and composition, heat and water will dislodge capsules from bacteria during laboratory procedures.

Principle

Crystal violet is applied as a stain. On application of 20% $CuSO_4$ solution, an osmotic difference is created due to which the stain diffuses towards the outer surface of the cell. This results in to appearance of a faint blue halo around a purple cell.

Materials Required

Slides, culture, inoculating loop, serum, 70% methanol, crystal violet, 20% $CuSO_4$, microscope, immersion oil.

Procedure

1. Transfer aseptically a loopful of serum on a clean and dry slide.
2. Mix it with loopful of culture.
3. Air dry the slides, but do not heat fix as this will distort the capsules.
4. Fix the smear with 1 or 2 drops of 70% V/V methanol or alcohol. Leave the alcohol on the smear for a minimum of 2 minutes or until the alcohol dries in the smear.
5. Flood the slide with crystal violet for 4-7 minutes.

6. Rinse slide thoroughly with 20% copper sulphate solution.
7. Dry and examine under oil immersion.

b) Observation of Capsular Staining

Observe your smear in the microscope under oil immersion and draw a few representative organisms from the smear below (use colour pencils):

Interpretation

The bacterial cell stains dark purple and capsule blue (mauve) colour.

Questions

Q1. What type of culture is used for demonstration of capsule-young or old and why?

Q2. Why is the smear not heat fixed?

Result

Date: Signature of Instructor

C) Spore Staining

Objective

1. To stain bacterial endospores.

Introduction

The term 'endospore' refers to the spore structure contained within a mother cell. The term 'spore' refers to the spore structure that exists free of the mother cell. Endospores may be located in the middle of the cells (central), at the end (terminal), or between the end and the middle of the cells (sub-terminal). The endospores themselves may be round or oval.

Endospore staining is a differential staining which stains bacterial endospores or spores. Some bacteria, including those belonging to the genera *Clostridium* and *Bacillus,* have the capacity to produce metabolically inactive cells called spores. Spores are highly resistant to hostile chemical and physical conditions and are produced by a process called sporulation, if environmental conditions become unfavorable for normal vegetative growth. The spore structures have a tough outer covering composed primarily of keratin which makes them resistant to heat, radiation, disinfectants, and desiccation. The bacteria will remain in this suspended state until conditions become favourable again and they can germinate and return to their vegetative state.

Principle

The primary stain in the endospore staining procedure is malachite green, which stains both vegetative cells and endospores. Heat is required to penetrate the endospore coat. Once the cells have cooled, the cells are decolorized with water, which selectively removes the malachite green from all vegetative cells but not from endospores. The counter stain then applied is safranin, which stains the decolorized vegetative cells pink. Thus, at the end of the staining procedure, the endospores are dark green, and vegetative cells are pink.

Materials Required

Slide, inoculating loop, culture, normal saline, malachite green, burner, safranin, microscope, immersion oil.

Procedure

1. Prepare a thin smear of the bacterial culture on a clean glass slide in normal saline solution.
2. Dry in air and fix over a flame.
3. Cover the slide with malachite green stain.
4. Heat the slide from below until the stain just begins to steam.
5. After approximately 5 minutes of steaming, wash the excess stain with water.
6. Flood the smear with safranin and stain for 1 minute.
7. Wash off the excess safranin with water, dry and observe using oil immersion.

Precautions

1. Do not allow malachite green to dry on slide during steaming.
2. Decolourization should be done only after cooling the slide.

Interpretation

The spores will stain green and vegetative cells red. Sometimes, the endospores don't take up the malachite green very well. In those cases, the endospores will appear as clear ovals or circles within a pink vegetative cell.

Questions

Q1. Why must heat be used with the application of the primary stain during endospore staining?

Q2. What advantage does the ability to sporulate give to pathogenic bacteria, such as *Clostridium tetani, Clostridium botulinum* and *Bacillus anthracis*?

c) Observation of Spore Staining

Observe your smear in the microscope under oil immersion and draw a few representative organisms from the smear below (use colour pencils):

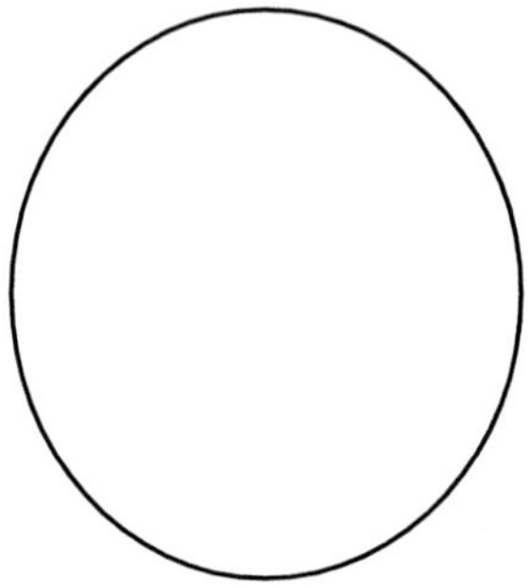

Result

Date: Signature of Instructor

Exercise **11**

Bacterial Motility

Objectives

1. To demonstrate motility of a given bacterial culture.
2. To learn about the different methods of motility determination.

Introduction

Motility of the bacteria is mediated by special structures called flagella. It occurs as a result of rotation of flagella in the way the shaft in electrical motor rotates. Bacteria normally move by run or swim and change direction by tumbling. Bacteria are observed for motility by different methods depending on the pathogenic capability of the organisms. For non-pathogens, slide techniques are used. The other methods to study bacterial motility are dark field microscopy and growing in semi-solid medium by stab method of inoculation (for pathogens).

Principle

Many bacteria in an aqueous environment appear to be moving erratically. This random motion of the water molecules bombarding the bacteria and causing them to move. Live, unstained, motile cells will demonstrate their motility under 40X magnification by displaying individual movement amongst cells which is unique and directional and much distinguished from the zig zag Brownian movement.

I.Hanging Drop Method

Bacterial motility can be demonstrated directly under the preparation. This is performed by examining a drop of organism suspension hanging from a cover slip in to the cavity of a slide.

Materials Required

Concavity/cavity slide, cover slip, liquid medium containing bacteria, petroleum jelly and microscope.

Procedure

1. Place a cover slip over a flat surface and put small amount of petroleum jelly on four corners of the cover slip.
2. Place a small drop of liquid medium containing bacteria at the centre of the cover slip.
3. Place a cavity slide over the cover slip in such a way that the concave surface is over the drop.
4. Gently reverse the slide. While reversing care should be taken not to disturb the hanging drop.
5. Focus the edge of the slide under high power (40X) and observe bacterial motility.

II.Wet Mount Slide

In a wet mount, the specimen is suspended in a drop of liquid (usually water), located between slide and cover glass. It is also sometimes referred as 'temporary mount' since it cannot be stored for long periods due to evaporation of liquid used. This method is mainly used for rapid investigations of non-pathogenic organisms.

Materials Required

Microscopic slides, cover slips, inoculating loop, micro pipette, Bunsen burner, young bacterial culture.

Procedure

1. Take a clean, scratch free glass slide.
2. Place 15-20 µl of the culture in the middle of the slide.
3. Lower a clean cover slip over the drop as though it were hinged at one side avoiding bubbles.
4. Examine the preparation under microscope first under 4x followed by 40X and 100X magnification.
5. Identify the motile organisms.

III.Soft Agar Stabbing (TUBE METHOD)

It is too dangerous to attempt to determine the motility of pathogenic micro organisms by slide techniques. A much safer method is to culture the organisms in a special medium that can demonstrate the presence of motility. The medium mainly used for this purpose is SIM medium (sulphide indole motility medium) which is a combination differential medium that tests three different parameters, sulphur reduction, indole production and motility. This media has a very soft consistency that allows motile bacteria to migrate readily through them causing cloudiness. The non-motile bacteria will only grow in the soft agar tube and only the area where they are inoculated. But in the case of motile bacteria, they will grow along the area of stab and will also swim out away from the stabbed area.

Materials Required

Test tube with SIM medium, inoculating straight wire/needle, young bacterial cultures.

Procedure

1. Flame and cool the inoculating needle and insert it in to the culture after flaming the neck of the tube.
2. Remove the cap from the tube of medium; flame the neck and stab it 2/3 of the way down to the bottom. Flame the neck of the tube again before returning the cap to the tube.
3. Incubate the tubes at room temperature for 24 to 48 hours.
4. Examine the growth after incubation.

Precautions

1. The bacteria are still alive in a hanging drop slide. Slides made from possible pathogens should be soaked in lysol for 5-10 minutes with the cover slip pulled aside to expose the drop before they are washed.
2. Always use a small drop of liquid medium and small amount of petroleum jelly.
3. Unstained bacteria are very transparent and difficult to see. Therefore, while focussing, reduce the lighting sufficiently to make the organisms visible.

Observation of Motility

Observe your slide in the microscope under 40X and draw a few representative motility patterns followed by the organisms:

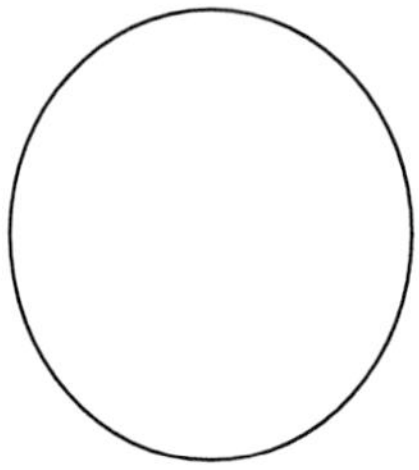

Questions

Q1. Why is petroleum jelly used in hanging drop method?

Q2. Why is a small drop of liquid medium used in hanging drop experiment?

Q3. Why a small amount of petroleum jelly is used in this experiment?

Q4. Why is the method named as "Hanging Drop'?

Q5. What type of culture is used for viewing motility-Young/old and why?

Q6. Why should we adjust and visualize the edge of the hanging drop to visualize the bacterial motility?

Result

Date: Signature of Instructor

Exercise 12

Culture Sensitivity Testing

Objective

1. To assess the *in vitro* antimicrobial sensitivity of a given bacterial culture.

Introduction

Antibiotic sensitivity is a term used to describe the susceptibility of bacteria to antibiotics. It is usually carried out to determine which antibiotic will be most successful in treating a bacterial infection *in vivo*. It is often done by Kirby-Bauer method (Disc diffusion method). Small discs containing antibiotics are placed on a plate upon which bacteria are growing. If the bacteria are sensitive to the antibiotic, a clear ring, or zone of inhibition is seen around the disc indicating poor growth.

Principle

The antibiotic-impregnated disc absorbs moisture from the agar and antibiotic diffuses into the agar medium. As the distance from the disc increases, there is a logarithmic reduction in the antibiotic concentration. The depth of the agar affects the extent of antimicrobial diffusion. Visible growth of bacteria occurs on the surface of the agar where the concentration of antibiotic has fallen below its inhibitory level for the test strain. The time required to reach the critical cell mass (4 to 10 h) is characteristic of each species but is influenced by medium composition and incubation time. The point at which the critical cell mass is reached appears as circle of bacterial growths, with the middle of the antibiotic disc forming the centre of the circle (zone of inhibition).

Materials Required

Test culture, Muller - Hinton agar, Brain Heart infusion (BHI) broth, 0.5 McFarland turbidity standard, sterile non-toxic cotton swabs, antibiotic discs and forceps.

McFarland 0.5 Turbidity standard

Solution A	(0.048 M $BaCl_2$)
$BaCl_2.H_2O$	1.175 g
Distilled water	100.000 ml
Solution B	(0.18 m H_2SO_4)
H_2SO_4	1.0 ml
Distilled water	100.0 ml
0.5 Standard	
Solution A	0.5 ml
Solution B	99.5 ml

Shake vigorously and dispense into 4-6 ml sealed tubes or screw-capped vials. Stored in the dark at room temperature and use upto 3 months. The turbidity standard should always be agitated before use.

Procedure

1. Selected 4-5 well-isolated and identical bacterial colonies grown overnight on a non-selective medium, such as Nutrient agar or Blood agar. Transfer these colonies into a tube of sterile BHI broth (5 ml).
2. Incubate the broth at 35-37^{0}C for 2-8 hours or until a light to moderate turbidity develops.

   Note : Alternatively the colonies may be directly suspended in sterile normal saline or BHI to prepare suspension of equivalent turbidity without incubation.
3. Compare the turbidity of the pre-incubated broth of the saline suspension of bacteria with 0.5. McFarland turbidity standard against a white background with contrasting black lines. Adjust the turbidity of the test suspension, if required with sterile broth or saline, until it equates to that of the turbidity standard. If turbidity is less, incubate the suspension for more duration.

4. Dip a sterile, non-toxic cotton swab on applicator stick into the standardised bacterial suspension and press excess fluid by pressing and rotating the swab against the inside wall of the tube.
5. Streak the swab in three directions over the entire surface of a sterile, dry plate of Mueller-Hinton agar, turning the plate at 60^0 angle between each streaking, so as to obtain a uniform growth.
6. Make a final sweep with the swab around the rim of the Petri dish.
7. Keep the plate at room temperature for 5-15 min to allow the excess moisture from the inoculums to be absorbed by the agar.
8. Place the antibiotic discs at equidistance (min 24 mm apart centre-to-centre) on to the agar surface using a sterile forceps or an antibiotic disc dispenser. Each disc should be gently pressed with the point of a sterile forceps.

   Note :

   a) Alter placing each disc sterilise the forceps in flame.

   b) Maximum 6 discs can be accommodated in a 9 cm. diameter Petri plate (24 mm apart).
9. Incubate the plate aerobically at 35-37^0 C in an inverted position for 16-18 hours or as recommended by the manufacture.
10. Read the diameter of zones of inhibition, around each disc from the back of the plate to the nearest mm using a ruler .The diameter of the zones should be read across the centre of the discs.

Precautions

a) The discs should be kept under appropriate conditions of temperature and moisture as mentioned by the manufacturer.

b) Discs that have passed the manufacturer's expiry date must be discarded.

c) The depth of agar in a Mueller-Hinton agar plate should be approximately 4 mm.

Observation of CST

Examine the BHI tubes for presence/absence of microbial growth and compare the turbidity with McFarland turbidity standard below:

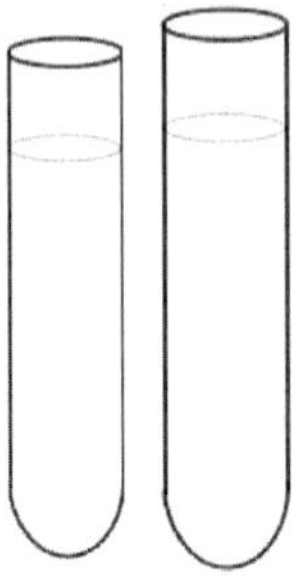

Observation of CST

Observe your slide in the microscope under 40X and draw a few representative organisms:

S.No.	Antibiotic	Symbol	Concen-tration	Zone of inhibition (in mm)	Interpretation (Refer standard Table as mentioned by manufacture)	Sensitive/ Resistant
1.						
2.						
3.						
4.						
5.						
6.						

Questions

Q1. What is the difference between bactericidal and bacteriostatic antibiotics?

Q2. Why do we use Mueller Hinton agar for antibiotic sensitivity test?

Result

Date: Signature of Instructor

□□□

Exercise **13**

Outlines of Collection, Transportation and Processing of Samples for Bacterial Disease Diagnosis

The purpose of a routine diagnostic laboratory is to provide a means for achieving a diagnosis as quickly as possible. In general, following points must be considered while collecting materials for laboratory diagnosis:

1. Full clinical history of the case should always accompany the samples. If available, a detailed postmortem report should also accompany the samples.
2. These sets of information will help the clinical microbiologist to select the most appropriate procedure and to furnish a meaningful interpretation of the results.
3. The nature of the specimen is determined by the clinical symptoms and history.

In bacteriology laboratory, samples are to be collected for three purposes:

1. Direct examination.
2. Isolation and identification of the infectious agent.
3. Serological investigation.

Collection of samples

1. Results of laboratory tests are directly dependent on the selection, mode of collection, preservation and shipment of the specimen.
2. Samples are to be collected and handled in a manner that will permit a high rate of recovery of the micro organisms present.

3. Samples are to be collected from typically affected animals.
4. When a herd is affected, it is desirable to send a typically infected animal to the laboratory so that laboratory personnel can collect blood and other samples before euthanasia.
5. Samples collected from a dead animal are of third choice.
6. In order to avoid failure of isolation of significant organisms, a wide range of tissues should be processed.
7. Always collect samples before treatment is started.
8. Collect specimens aseptically during the early acute phase.
9. Obtain a tentative diagnosis from veterinarian who has collected the sample.

Specimens for Diagnosis of Becterial Infections

Blood

- Clean the area thoroughly with 70% alcohol. Collect blood aseptically and inoculate directly into Brain Heart Infusion broth (BHI) and Fluid thioglycolate (FTG) broth.
- Incubate for 24 to 48 hours aerobically (BHI) and anaerobically (FTG)and subculture on blood agar.
- Prepare blood smears at the time of collection of blood and examine them.

Cerebrospinal fluid

- Collect one ml of CSF aseptically from the lumbosacral area and inoculate as for blood.

Specimens in eye infections

- Collect the specimens on dry cotton swabs and inoculate immediately on to solid medium.

Specimens in ear infections

- Collect the specimens on dry cotton swabs and inoculate directly on to solid media and incubate aerobically and anaerobically.

Urine

- Collect mid stream urine by catheterization. Inoculate on to suitable media with or without centrifugation.
- If transportation is required, add boric acid at the rate of 0.5 g to 28 ml of urine.

Faeces

- Take rectal swabs and inoculate on to blood agar and Mac Conkey's agar and incubate aerobically and anaerobically.
- If *Salmonella* is suspected, inoculate in selenite broth, incubate for 6 to 8 hours , and subculture on MacConkey's agar or Brilliant green agar.
- If required, transport the faecal material in equal quantity of phosphate buffer and glycerol at pH 7.

Milk

- Collect mid stream milk aseptically from each teat into sterile bottles and inoculate onto solid media.

Serous cavity fluid

- Follow the same procedure as for cerebrospinal fluid.

Cervical and uterine discharges

- Take special care to avoid contamination. Collect by catheter or washings and inoculate onto solid media and incubate aerobically, anaerobically and under increased carbon dioxide tension.
- When cervical or vaginal swabs are collected, they are to be immediately placed in the transport medium (nutrient broth) to avoid drying.

Prepucial washings and semen

- Collect prepucial washings and semen, aseptically, if genital infections are suspected in male animals.

Pus

- Collect pus from the deep region of the wound with a sterile swab after cleaning the wound surface with 70% alcohol.

Samples to be collected at the time of postmortem

- Collect the specimens as early as possible after death.
- Collect pieces of vital organs aseptically and place them in a sterile vials.
- In reproductive problems, collect uterine discharges.
- Placenta and aborted foetus should be collected.
- If intestinal disorders are suspected, collect intestinal contents.
- From decomposed carcasses, isolation of specific bacterial organisms can be attempted from the bone marrow of long bones.

Specimens for Diagnosis of Fungal Infections

Blood

- Collect blood aseptically into bottles containing anticoagulant.

Hair

- Collect hair (pluck) from animals suspected for dermatophytosis.
- Obtain at least 10 to 15 hairs and place them in wide mouthed bottles.

Nails or hooves

- Collect nails or hooves from animals suspected for infections with dermatophytes, *Candida*, *Fusarium*, etc.
- Wipe the nails or hooves thoroughly with 70% alcohol. Scrape the under surface, if it appears to be infected.

Skin

- Collect skin from animals believed to be suffering from dermatophytosis or cutaneous candidiasis.

- After sterilizing the lesion area, scrape the lesion with a sterile scalpel or razor blade.
- Make sure to scrape the peripheral area of the lesion, where viable mycotic agent will be found.

Urine

1. Collect and examine urine when animals are suspected for candidiasis.
2. Agents of, blastomycosis, cryptococcosis, etc. can also be seen in urine.
3. Early morning samples are best, as the organisms will multiply overnight producing higher yeast count, assuring their isolation.

Milk

- Collect milk separately from different quarters, aseptically, after washing with mild disinfectant.

Aborted materials

- Collect aseptically, foetal stomach contents, peritoneal fluid, foetal liver and spleen, placenta and uterine discharge, and send to the laboratory through a special messenger.

Body fluids

- Aspirate aseptically from joints and body cavities.

Cerebrospinal fluid

- Collected primarily for the isolation of *Cryptococcus neoformans*.
- Send the aseptically collected CSF to the laboratory immediately.
- Store in the refrigerator, if there is a delay of 1 hour (but not more than one hour).

Preservation of specimens

1. All materials should reach the laboratory at the earliest and not later than 6 hours after collection.

2. This period, if required can be extended up to 18 hours, due to delay in transit, if the materials are well packed, labelled, and kept at 2 to 10°C.
3. Wet ice is preferred for materials intended for bacteriological examination.
4. Specimens must be kept cold unless they can reach the laboratory within an hour after collection.
5. In general, they must be stored frozen (-20°C) or kept at 4°C if examined within 24 hours.

Transport of specimens serum sample for serological studies

1. Specimens are transported to the laboratory in insulated containers. Wide mouthed corked glass containers are suitable.
2. Cotton plugged tubes are unacceptable. All containers must be labelled.
3. It is also advantageous, if the inner container is carefully wrapped in absorbent paper or other such material to absorb shock and any fluid that may be spilt.
4. It is preferable to collect paired serum samples (one during the acute phase of the illness and the other during the convalescent phase [14 to 21 days]).
5. To collect serum, draw blood from the jugular vein (large animals), wing vein (chicken), or saphenous vein (dogs). Do not freeze the blood.
6. Allow it to form the clot. Incubate at 37°C for 30 minutes and then transfer to 4°C.
7. Retraction of the clot occurs and serum is usually expressed in 12 to 18 hours.
8. If not, centrifuge at 1, 000 rpm for 10 minutes to separate serum. Merthiolate (at a strength of 1 :10000) may be added as a preservative.
9. Transfer the serum to screw capped vials, seal and store at -20°C till used.

❑❑❑

Exercise 14

Characterization of Staphylococcus, Streptococcus, *E. coli*, Salmonella, Klebsiella and Proteus, Pseudomonas, Pasteurella and Clostridium

Staphylococcus

I. Etiologic agent

II. Classification

1	Domain
2	Phylum
3	Class
4	Order
5	Family
6	Genus

III. Sample Collection (from live and dead animal)

IV. Laboratory Diagnosis

A) Direct Examination of the Specimen

B) Isolation and Identification of the agent

C) Pathogenicity test

D) Molecular Identification

E) Serology

A) Direct Examination of the Specimen

i) Staining method

Morphology by staining

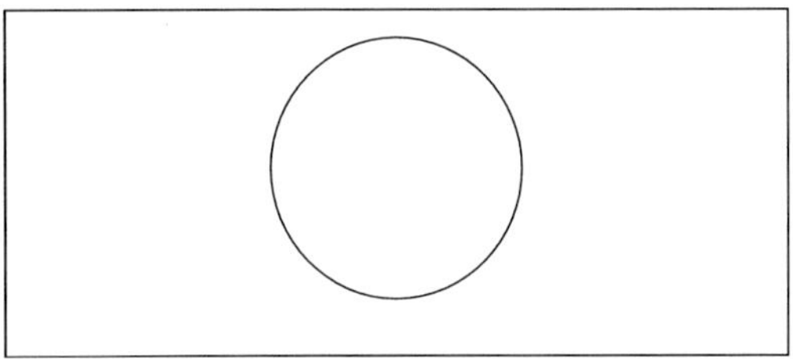

ii) Immunological method

iii) Nucleic acid method by direct sample

B) Isolation and Identification of the agent

i) Isolation of the agent

1. Basal/enriched media ______________________________

2. Selective/Differential media __________________________

ii) Identification of the agent

1. Staining method ____________________________________

Morphology

____

____

____

____

____

____

2. Colony characteristics in media

SOLID MEDIUM		LIQUID MEDIUM	
Shape		Degree of growth	
Size		Turbidity	
Elevation		Surface growth	
Surface		Odour	
Edge			
Opacity			
Color			
Emulsifiability			

Growth in Media

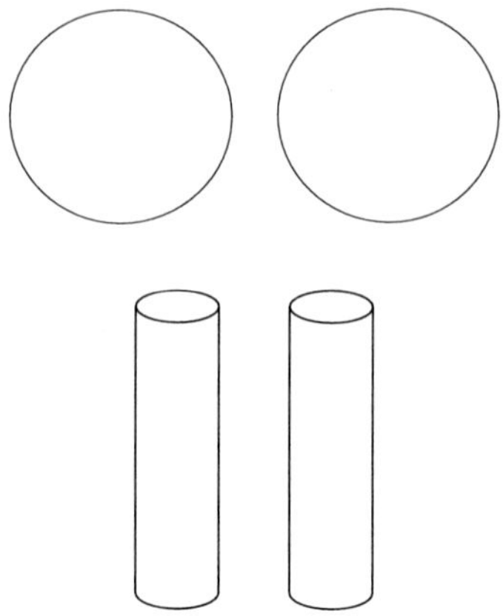

3. Biochemical characteristics

CARBOHYDRATE FERMENTATION TES T			
Arabinose		Inuline	
Dextrin		Mannose	
Dulcitol		Mannitol	
Fructose		Maltose	
Glucose		Salicin	
Glycerol		Sorbitol	
OTHER BIOCHEMICAL TEST			
Indole		Urease	
Methyl Red		H_2S production	
Voges Proskaur		Aesculine Hydrolysis	
Citrate			
Catalase			
Oxidase			
Nitrate			

4. Immunological/Antigen detection (Serotyping)

5. Nucleic acid method

C) Pathogenicity test - Animal Inoculation (name of the lab animal, route of inoculation and its outcome)

D) Molecular Identification

E) Serology

Q1. What do you understand by hot-cold lysis?

Q2. What is the difference between serum and plasma? How will you prepare plasma?

Q3. For the preparation of blood agar media, why do we not collect the sterile blood by adding anti-coagulant in the flask?

Q4. Differentiate between staphylococci and streptococci in tabulated form?

Date: Signature of Instructor

Streptococcus

I. Etiolofic agent ____________________

II. Classification

1	Domain
2	Phylum
3	Class
4	Order
5	Family
6	Genus

III. Sample Collection (from live and dead animal)

____

____

____

____

____

IV. Laboratory Diagnosis

A) Direct Examination of the Specimen

B) Isolation and Identification of the agent

C) Pathogenicity test

D) Molecular Identification

E) Serology

A) Direct Examination of the Specimen

i) Staining method

____

____

____

____

Morphology by staining

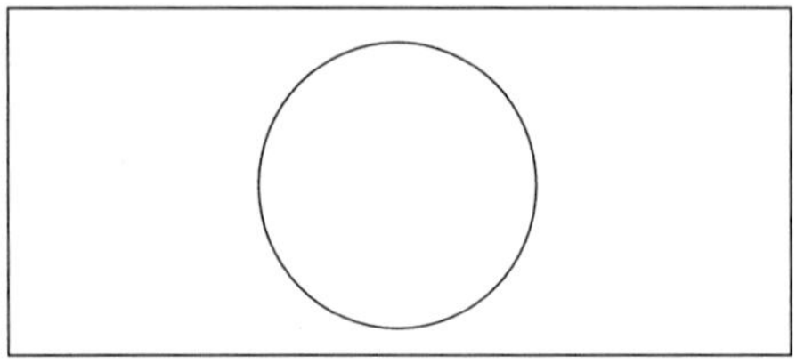

ii) Immunological method

iii) Nucleic acid method by direct sample

B) Isolation and Identification of the agent

i) Isolation of the agent

1. Basal/enriched media ______
2. Selective / Differential media ______

ii) Identification of the agent

1. Staining method ______

Morphology

____

____

____

____

____

____

____

2. Colony characteristics in media

SOLID MEDIUM		**LIQUID MEDIUM**	
Shape		Degree of growth	
Size		Turbidity	
Elevation		Surface growth	
Surface		Odour	
Edge			
Opacity			
Colour			
Emulsifiability			

Growth in Media

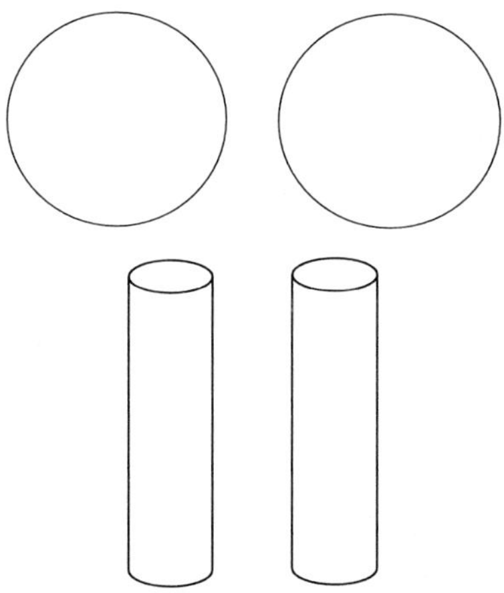

3. Biochemical characteristics

CARBOHYDRATE FERMENTATION TEST			
Arabinose		Inuline	
Dextrin		Mannose	
Dulcitol		Mannitol	
Fructose		Maltose	
Glucose		Salicin	
Glycerol		Sorbitol	
OTHER BIOCHEMICAL TEST			
Indole		Urease	
Methyl Red		H_2S production	
Voges Proskaur		Aesculine Hydrolysis	
Citrate			
Catalase			
Oxidase			
Nitrate			

4. Immunological/Antigen detection (Serotyping) –

____

____

____

____

____

____

5. Nucleic acid method

____

____

____

____

____

____

C) Pathogenicity test - Animal Inoculation (name of the lab animal, route of inoculation and its outcome)

D) Molecular Method

E) Serology

Q1. What is plasmodesma? Explain.

Q2. Why are streptococci found in chains?

Q3. Write the principle of CAMP test and explain diagrammatically.

Q4. What type of haemolysis is produced by *Streptococcus pyogenes* on blood agar plate? Explain diagrammatically.

Date: Signature of Instructor

E. Coli

I. Etiologic agent ______________________________

II. Classification

1	Domain	
2	Phylum	
3	Class	
4	Order	
5	Family	
6	Genus	

III. Sample Collection (from live and dead animal)

____

____

____

____

____

IV. Laboratory diagnosis

A) Direct Examination of the Specimen
B) Isolation and Identification of the agent
C) Pathogenicity test
D) Molecular Identification
E) Serology

A) Direct Examination of the Specimen

i) Staining method

____

____

____

____

____

Morphology by staining

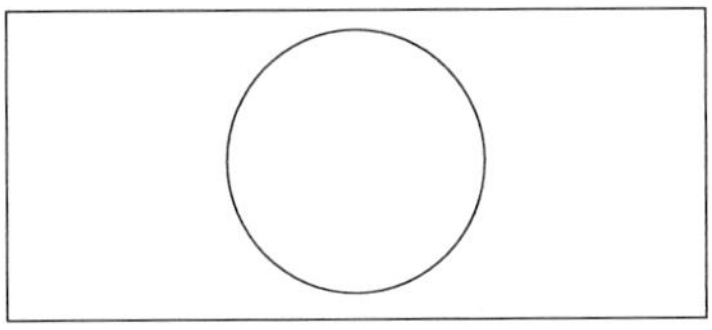

ii) Immunological method

iii) Nucleic acid method by direct sample

B) Isolation and Identification of the agent

i) Isolation of the agent

1. Basal/enriched media __________

2. Selective/Differential media __________

ii) Identification of the agent

1. Staining method __________

Morphology

2. Colony characteristics in media

SOLID MEDIUM		LIQUID MEDIUM	
Shape		Degree of growth	
Size		Turbidity	
Elevation		Surface growth	
Surface		Odour	
Edge			
Opacity			
Colour			
Emulsifiability			

Growth in Media

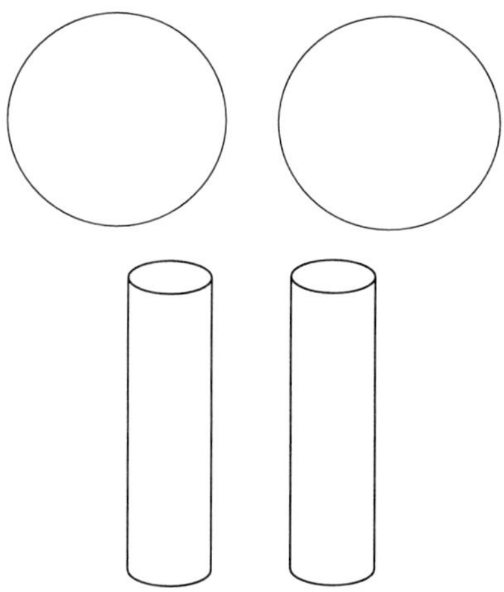

3. Biochemical characteristics

CARBOHYDRATE FERMENTATION TEST			
Arabinose		Inuline	
Dextrin		Mannose	
Dulcitol		Mannitol	
Fructose		Maltose	
Glucose		Salicin	
Glycerol		Sorbitol	

OTHER BIOCHEMICAL TEST			
Indole		Urease	
Methyl Red		H_2S production	
Voges Proskaur		Aesculine Hydrolysis	
Citrate			
Catalase			
Oxidase			
Nitrate			

4. Immunological/Antigen detection (Serotyping)

5. Nucleic acid method

C) Pathogenicity test - Animal Inoculation (name of the lab animal, route of inoculation and its outcome)

D) Molecular Method

E) Serology

____

____

____

____

Q1. Write the mechanism as to why metallic sheen is produced by *E.coli* on EMB plate?

Q2. Write the name of indicator(s) present in MLA, EMB and citrate agar. What colour these indicators produce in acidic and alkaline medium?

Q3. Write the name of various genera of Enterobacteriaceae family.

Q4. How will you isolate and identify *E. coli* from the faeces of bird?

Date: Signature of Instructor

Salmonella

I. Etiologic agent ______________________________

II. Classification

1	Domain	
2	Phylum	
3	Class	
4	Order	
5	Family	
6	Genus	

III. Sample Collection (from live and dead animal)

____

____

____

____

IV. Laboratory Diagnosis

A) Direct Examination of the Specimen

B) Isolation and Identification of the agent

C) Pathogenicity test

D) Molecular Identification

E) Serology

A) Direct Examination of the Specimen

i) Staining method

____

____

____

____

____

Morphology by staining

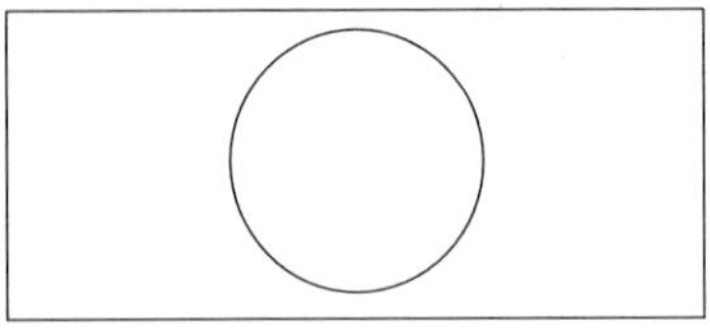

ii) Immunological method

iii) Nucleic acid method by direct sample

B) Isolation and Identification of the agent:

i) Isolation of the agent

1. Basal/enriched media ____________

2. Selective/Differential media ____________

ii) Identification of the agent

1. Staining method ____________

Morphology

2. Colony characteristics in media

SOLID MEDIUM		LIQUID MEDIUM	
Shape		Degree of growth	
Size		Turbidity	
Elevation		Surface growth	
Surface		Odour	
Edge			
Opacity			
Colour			
Emulsifiability			

Growth in Media

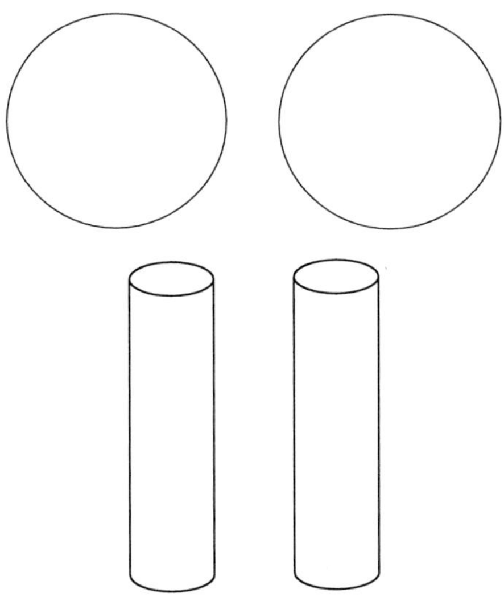

3. Biochemical characteristics

CARBOHYDRATE FERMENTATION TEST			
Arabinose		Inuline	
Dextrin		Mannose	
Dulcitol		Mannitol	
Fructose		Maltose	
Glucose		Salicin	
Glycerol		Sorbitol	
OTHER BIOCHEMICAL TEST			
Indole		Urease	
Methyl Red		H_2S production	
Voges Proskaur		Aesculine Hydrolysis	
Citrate			
Catalase			
Oxidase			
Nitrate			

4. Immunological/Antigen detection (Serotyping)

5. Nucleic acid method

C) Pathogenicity test - Animal Inoculation (name of the lab animal, route of inoculation and its outcome)

D) Molecular Method

E) Serology

Q1. Write briefly the Kauffman and White scheme of classification of *Salmonella.*

Q2. Explain Vi antigen.

Q3. Write three selective media for *Salmonella.*

Q4. Write the role of indicator in the media used for isolation and identification of members of family Enterobacteriaceae.

Q5. Define 'O' and 'H' antigens of *Salmonella.*

Q6. Differentiate *Klebsiella* pneumonia from *E.coli, Proteus* and *Salmonella* organisms with respect to their morphology culture and biochemical characteristics. Give your answer in tabulated form only.

Properties	*E.coli*	*K.pneumoniae*	Proteus	Salmonella
Morphology				
Cultural Characters				
Biochemical Characters				

Date: Signature of Instructor

Klebsiella

I. Etiologic agent ____________________

II. Classification

1 Domain
2 Phylum
3 Class
4 Order
5 Family
6 Genus

III. Sample Collection (from live and dead animal)

IV. Laboratory diagnosis

A) Direct Examination of the Specimen
B) Isolation and Identification of the agent
C) Pathogenicity test
D) Molecular Identification
E) Serology

A) Direct Examination of the Specimen

i) Staining method

Morphology by staining

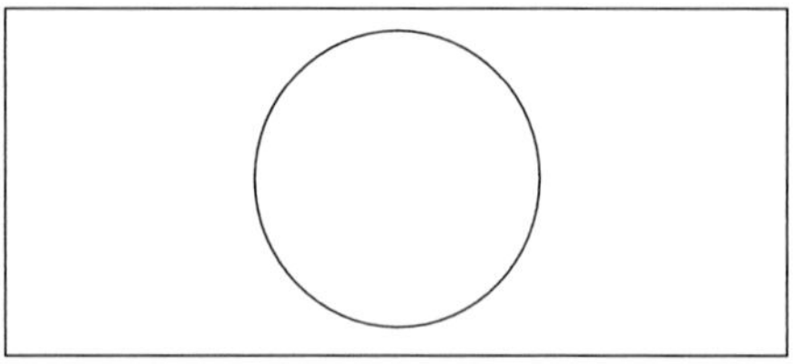

ii) Immunological method

iii) Nucleic acid method by direct sample

B) Isolation and Identification of the agent

i) Isolation of the agent

1. Basal/Enriched media
2. Selective/Differential media

ii) Identification of the agent

1. Staining method

Morphology

____

____

____

____

____

2. Colony characteristics in media

SOLID MEDIUM		**LIQUID MEDIUM**	
Shape		Degree of growth	
Size		Turbidity	
Elevation		Surface growth	
Surface		Odour	
Edge			
Opacity			
Colour			
Emulsifiability			

Growth in Media

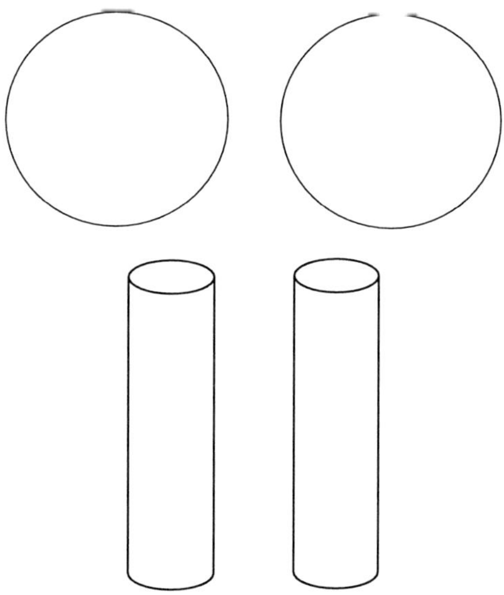

3. Biochemical characteristics

CARBOHYDRATE FERMENTATION TEST			
Arabinose		Inuline	
Dextrin		Mannose	
Dulcitol		Mannitol	
Fructose		Maltose	
Glucose		Salicin	
Glycerol		Sorbitol	

4. Immunological/Antigen detection (Serotyping)

5. Nucleic acid method

C) Pathogenicity test - Animal Inoculation (name of the lab animal, route of inoculation and its outcome)

D) Molecular Method

E) Serology

Date: Signature of Instructor

Proteus

I. Etiologic agent ______________________________

II. Classification

1	Domain
2	Phylum
3	Class
4	Order
5	Family
6	Genus

III. Sample Collection (from live and dead animal)

____

____

____

____

IV. Laboratory diagnosis

A) Direct Examination of the Specimen

B) Isolation and Identification of the agent

C) Pathogenicity test

D) Molecular Identification

E) Serology

A) Direct Examination of the Specimen

i) Staining method

____

____

____

____

Morphology by staining

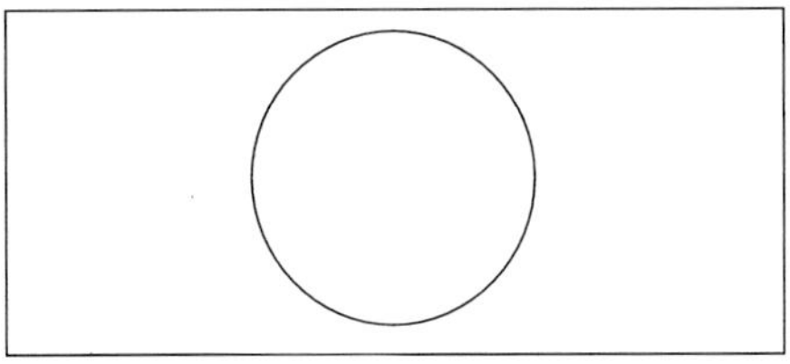

ii) Immunological method

iii) Nucleic acid method by direct sample

B) Isolation and Identification of the agent

i) Isolation of the agent

1. Basal/Enriched media

2. Selective/Differential media

ii) Identification of the agent

1. Staining method

Morphology

2. Colony characteristics in media

SOLID MEDIUM		LIQUID MEDIUM	
Shape		Degree of growth	
Size		Turbidity	
Elevation		Surface growth	
Surface		Odour	
Edge			
Opacity			
Colour			
Emulsifiability			

Growth in Media

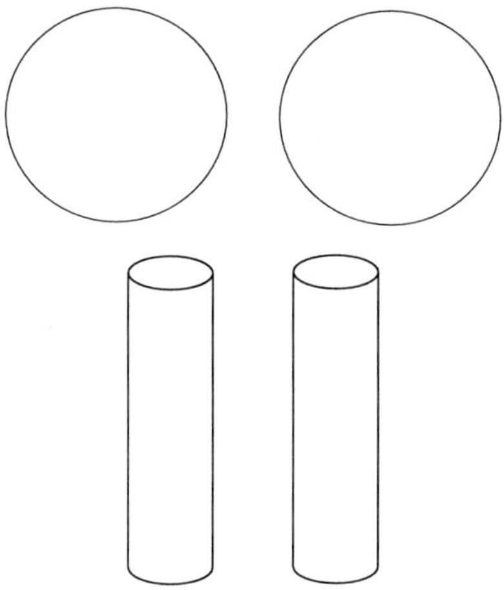

3. Biochemical characteristics

CARBOHYDRATE FERMENTATION TEST			
Arabinose		Inuline	
Dextrin		Mannose	
Dulcitol		Mannitol	
Fructose		Maltose	
Glucose		Salicin	
Glycerol		Sorbitol	

OTHER BIOCHEMICAL TEST			
Indole		Urease	
Methyl Red		H_2S production	
Voges Proskaur		Aesculine Hydrolysis	
Citrate			
Catalase			
Oxidase			
Nitrate			

4. Immunological/Antigen detection (Serotyping)

5. Nucleic acid method

C) Pathogenicity test - Animal Inoculation (name of the lab animal, route of inoculation and its outcome)

D) Molecular Method

E) Serology

Date: Signature of Instructor

Pseudomonas

I. Etiologic agent ______________________

II. Classification

1	Domain
2	Phylum
3	Class
4	Order
5	Family
6	Genus

III. Sample Collection (from live and dead animal)

____

____

____

____

____

IV. Laboratory diagnosis

A) Direct Examination of the Specimen

B) Isolation and Identification of the agent

C) Pathogenicity test

D) Molecular Identification

E) Serology

A) Direct Examination of the Specimen

i) Staining method

____

____

____

____

____

Morphology by staining

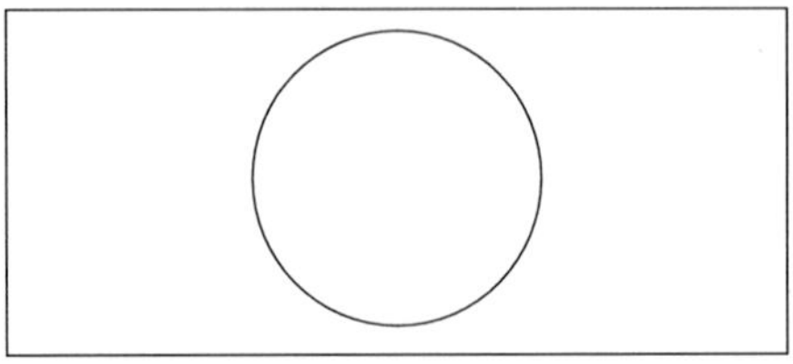

ii) Immunological method

iii) Nucleic acid method by direct sample

B) Isolation and Identification of the agent

i) Isolation of the agent

   1. Basal/Enriched media

   2. Selective/Differential media

ii) Identification of the agent

1. Staining method

Morphology

2. Colony characteristics in media

SOLID MEDIUM		**LIQUID MEDIUM**	
Shape		Degree of growth	
Size		Turbidity	
Elevation		Surface growth	
Surface		Odour	
Edge			
Opacity			
Colour			
Emulsifiability			

Growth in Media

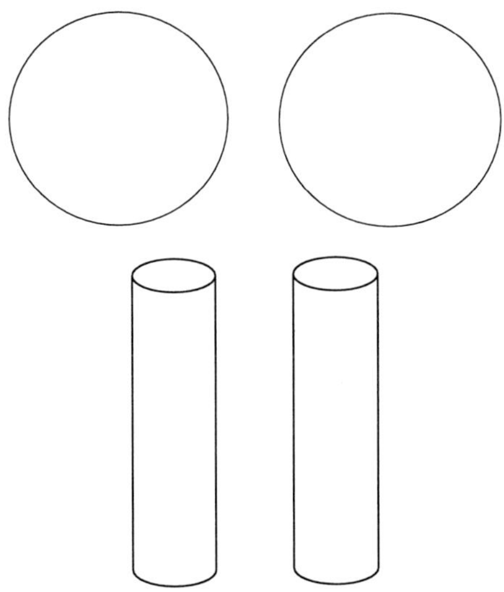

3. Biochemical characteristics

CARBOHYDRATE FERMENTATION TEST			
Arabinose		Inuline	
Dextrin		Mannose	
Dulcitol		Mannitol	
Fructose		Maltose	
Glucose		Salicin	
Glycerol		Sorbitol	
OTHER BIOCHEMICAL TEST			
Indole		Urease	
Methyl Red		H_2S production	
Voges Proskaur		Aesculine Hydrolysis	
Citrate			
Catalase			
Oxidase			
Nitrate			

4. Immunological/Antigen detection (Serotyping)

5. Nucleic acid method

C) Pathogenicity test - Animal Inoculation (name of the lab animal, route of inoculation and its outcome)

D) Molecular Method

E) Serology

Date: Signature of Instructor

Pasteurella

I. Etiologic agent ___________________________

II. Classification

1	Domain	
2	Phylum	
3	Class	
4	Order	
5	Family	
6	Genus	

III. Sample Collection (from live and dead animal)

IV. Laboratory diagnosis

A) Direct Examination of the Specimen
B) Isolation and Identification of the agent
C) Pathogenicity test
D) Molecular Identification
E) Serology

A) Direct Examination of the Specimen

i) Staining method

Morphology by staining

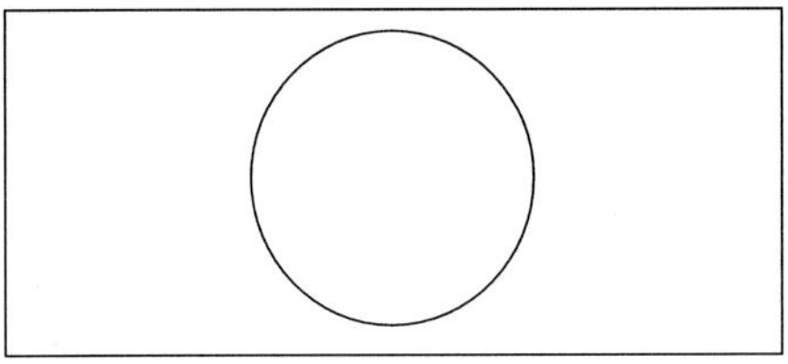

ii) Immunological method

iii) Nucleic acid method by direct sample

B) Isolation and Identification of the agent

i) Isolation of the agent

1. Basal/Enriched media

2. Selective/Differential media

ii) Identification of the agent

1. Staining method

Morphology

2. Colony characteristics in media

SOLID MEDIUM		LIQUID MEDIUM	
Shape		Degree of growth	
Size		Turbidity	
Elevation		Surface growth	
Surface		Odour	
Edge			
Opacity			
Colour			
Emulsifiability			

Growth in Media

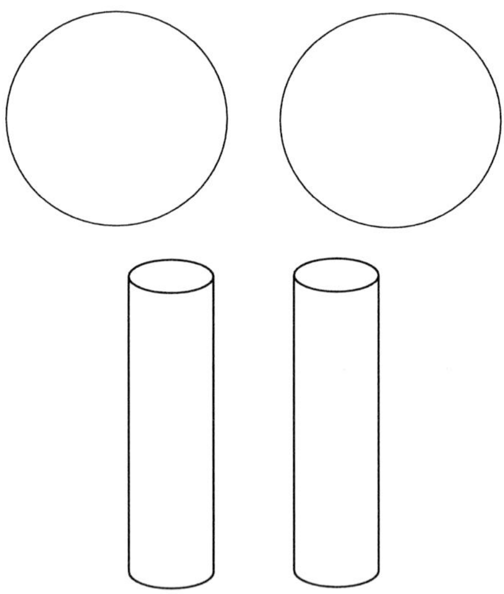

3. Biochemical characteristics

CARBOHYDRATE FERMENTATION TEST			
Arabinose		Inuline	
Dextrin		Mannose	
Dulcitol		Mannitol	
Fructose		Maltose	
Glucose		Salicin	
Glycerol		Sorbitol	
OTHER BIOCHEMICAL TEST			
Indole		Urease	
Methyl Red		H_2S production	
Voges Proskaur		Aesculine Hydrolysis	
Citrate			
Catalase			
Oxidase			
Nitrate			

4. Immunological/Antigen detection (Serotyping)

____

____

____

____

5. Nucleic acid method

____

____

____

____

____

C) Pathogenicity test - Animal Inoculation (name of the lab animal, route of inoculation and its outcome)

D) Molecular Method

E) Serology

Q1. What do you understand by bipolar staining?

Q2. Enlist diseases caused by pasteurella organism.

Date: Signature of Instructor

Clostridium

I. Etiologic agent ____________________

II. Classification

1	Domain	
2	Phylum	
3	Class	
4	Order	
5	Family	
6	Genus	

III. Sample Collection (from live and dead animal)

____

____

____

____

____

IV. Laboratory diagnosis

A) Direct Examination of the Specimen

B) Isolation and Identification of the agent

C) Pathogenicity test

D) Molecular Identification

E) Serology

A) Direct Examination of the Specimen

i) Staining method

____

____

____

____

Morphology by staining

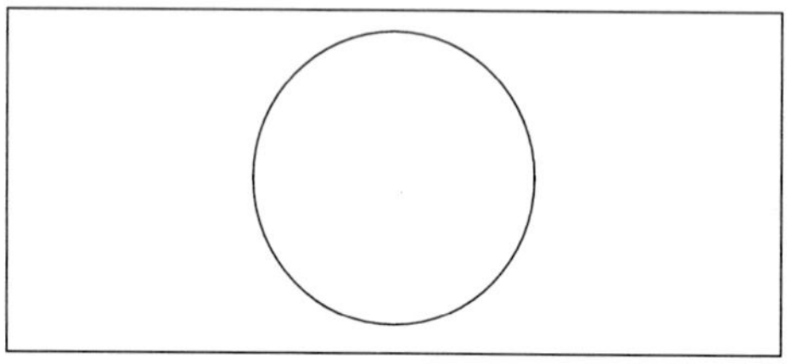

ii) Immunological method

iii) Nucleic acid method by direct sample

B) Isolation and Identification of the agent

i) Isolation of the agent

1. Basal/Enriched media

2. Selective/Differential media

ii) Identification of the agent

1. Staining method

Morphology

2. Colony characteristics in media

SOLID MEDIUM		LIQUID MEDIUM	
Shape		Degree of growth	
Size		Turbidity	
Elevation		Surface growth	
Surface		Odour	
Edge			
Opacity			
Colour			
Emulsifiability			

Growth in Media

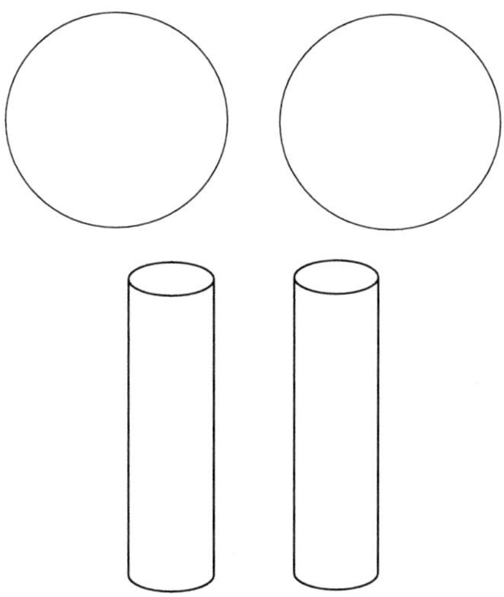

3. Biochemical characteristics

CARBOHYDRATE FERMENTATION TEST			
Arabinose		Inuline	
Dextrin		Mannose	
Dulcitol		Mannitol	
Fructose		Maltose	
Glucose		Salicin	
Glycerol		Sorbitol	
OTHER BIOCHEMICAL TEST			
Indole		Urease	
Methyl Red		H_2S production	
Voges Proskaur		Aesculine Hydrolysis	
Citrate			
Catalase			
Oxidase			
Nitrate			

4. Immunological/Antigen detection (Serotyping)

5. Nucleic acid method

C) Pathogenicity test - Animal Inoculation (name of the lab animal, route of inoculation and its outcome)

D) Molecular Method

E) Serology

Q1. Why is Robertson cooked meat medium advantageous for the growth of *Clostridium* species?

Q2. Write the species of *Clostridium* that produces central and sub-terminal spores.

Q3. Describe various toxins of *Clostridium perfringens*.

Q4. Which type of *Clostridium perfringens* produces enterotoxins? Write its molecular weight.

Q5. Draw the diagram of various types of spores produced by *Clostridium* species.

Q6. Name the species of *Clostridium* that are capsulated.

Q7. Write the various toxins of *Clostridium chauvoei*.

Date: Signature of Instructor

❑❑❑

Exercise **15**

Isolation and Identification of Bacteria from Clinical Cases of Mastitis, Abortions, Enteric, Respiratory & Pyogenic Infections

Mastitis

I. Etiologic agent ________________________________

II. Classification

1	Domain	
2	Phylum	
3	Class	
4	Order	
5	Family	
6	Genus	

III. Sample Collection (from live and dead animal)

____

____

____

____

____

IV. Laboratory diagnosis

A) Direct Examination of the Specimen

B) Isolation and Identification of the agent

C) Pathogenicity test

D) Molecular Identification

E) Serology

A) Direct Examination of the Specimen

i) Staining method

Morphology by staining

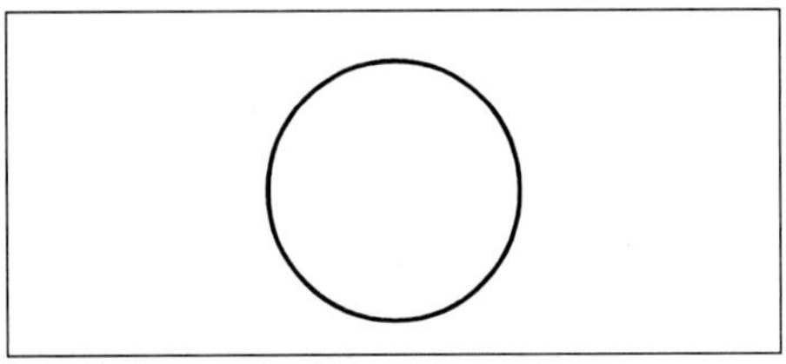

ii) Immunological method

iii) Nucleic acid method by direct sample

B) Isolation and Identification of the agent

i) Isolation of the agent -

1. Basal/Enriched media ______________________

2. Selective/Differential media ______________________

ii) Identification of the agent

1. Staining method ______________________

Morphology

____

____

____

____

____

____

____

2. Colony characteristics in media

SOLID MEDIUM		**LIQUID MEDIUM**	
Shape		Degree of growth	
Size		Turbidity	
Elevation		Surface growth	
Surface		Odour	
Edge			
Opacity			
Colour			
Emulsifiability			

Growth in Media

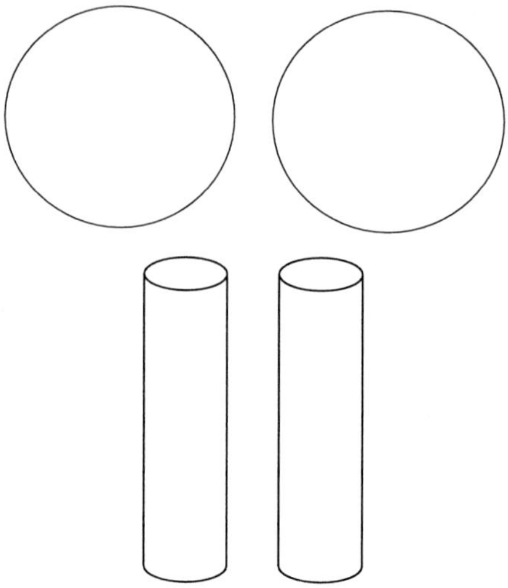

3. Biochemical characteristics

CARBOHYDRATE FERMENTATION TEST			
Arabinose		Inuline	
Dextrin		Mannose	
Dulcitol		Mannitol	
Fructose		Maltose	
Glucose		Salicin	
Glycerol		Sorbitol	
OTHER BIOCHEMICAL TEST			
Indole		Urease	
Methyl Red		H_2S production	
Voges Proskaur		Aesculine Hydrolysis	
Citrate			
Catalase			
Oxidase			
Nitrate			

4. Immunological/Antigen detection (Serotyping)

5. Nucleic acid method

C. Pathogenicity test - Animal Inoculation (name of the lab animal, route of inoculation and its outcome)

D. Molecular Method

E. Serology

Mastitis

I. Etiologic agent ____________________

II. Classification

1	Domain	
2	Phylum	
3	Class	
4	Order	
5	Family	
6	Genus	

III. Sample Collection (from live and dead animal)

IV. LABORATORY DIAGNOSIS

A) Direct Examination of the Specimen

B) Isolation and Identification of the agent

C) Pathogenicity test

D) Molecular Identification

E) Serology

A) Direct Examination of the Specimen

i) Staining method

Morphology by staining

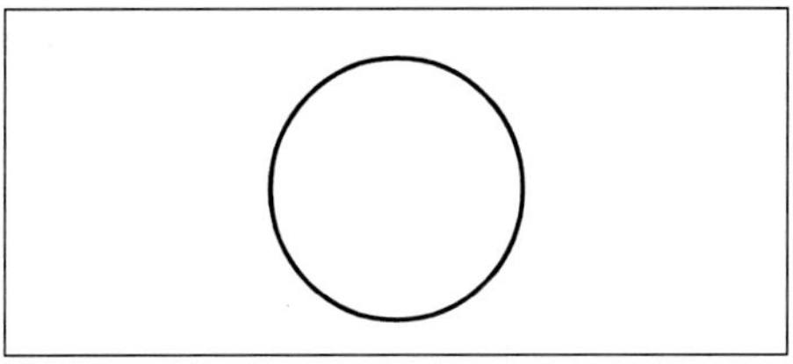

ii) Immunological method

iii) Nucleic acid method by direct sample

B) Isolation and Identification of the agent

i) Isolation of the agent

1. Basal/Enriched media

2. Selective/Differential media

ii) Identification of the agent

1. Staining method

Morphology

2. Colony characteristics in media

SOLID MEDIUM		LIQUID MEDIUM	
Shape		Degree of growth	
Size		Turbidity	
Elevation		Surface growth	
Surface		Odour	
Edge			
Opacity			
Colour			
Emulsifiability			

Growth in Media

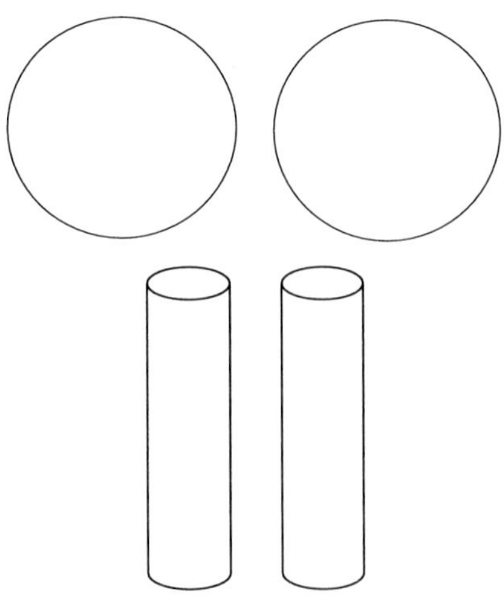

3. Biochemical characteristics

CARBOHYDRATE FERMENTATION TEST			
Arabinose		Inuline	
Dextrin		Mannose	
Dulcitol		Mannitol	
Fructose		Maltose	
Glucose		Salicin	
Glycerol		Sorbitol	
OTHER BIOCHEMICAL TEST			
Indole		Urease	
Methyl Red		H_2S production	
Voges Proskaur		Aesculine Hydrolysis	
Citrate			
Catalase			
Oxidase			
Nitrate			

4. Immunological/Antigen detection (Serotyping)

____

____

____

____

____

5. Nucleic acid method

____

____

____

____

____

C. Pathogenicity test - Animal Inoculation (name of the lab animal, route of inoculation and its outcome)

D. Molecular Method

E. Serology

Mastitis

I. Etiologic agent ____________________

II. Classification

1	Domain	
2	Phylum	
3	Class	
4	Order	
5	Family	
6	Genus	

III. Sample Collection (from live and dead animal)

____

____

____

____

IV. Laboratory diagnosis

A) Direct Examination of the Specimen

B) Isolation and Identification of the agent

C) Pathogenicity test

D) Molecular Identification

E) Serology

A) Direct Examination of the Specimen

i) Staining method

____

____

____

____

____

Morphology by staining

ii) Immunological method

____

____

____

____

____

iii) Nucleic acid method by direct sample

____

____

____

____

____

B) Isolation and Identification of the agent

i) Isolation of the agent

1. Basal/Enriched media ________________________

2. Selective/Differential media ____________________

ii) Identification of the agent

1. Staining method ____________________________

Morphology

____

____

____

____

____

2. Colony characteristics in media

SOLID MEDIUM		**LIQUID MEDIUM**	
Shape		Degree of growth	
Size		Turbidity	
Elevation		Surface growth	
Surface		Odour	
Edge			
Opacity			
Colour			
Emulsifiability			

Growth in Media

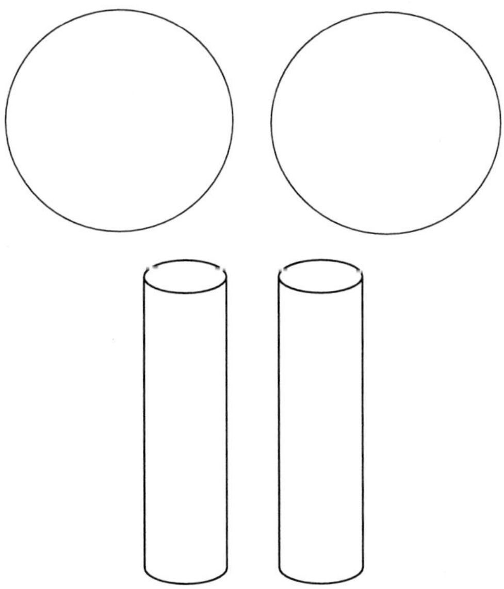

3. Biochemical characteristics

CARBOHYDRATE FERMENTATION TEST			
Arabinose		Inuline	
Dextrin		Mannose	
Dulcitol		Mannitol	
Fructose		Maltose	
Glucose		Salicin	
Glycerol		Sorbitol	
OTHER BIOCHEMICAL TEST			
Indole		Urease	
Methyl Red		H_2S production	
Voges Proskaur		Aesculine Hydrolysis	
Citrate			
Catalase			
Oxidase			
Nitrate			

4. Immunological/Antigen detection (Serotyping)

5. Nucleic acid method

C. Pathogenicity test - Animal Inoculation (name of the lab animal, route of inoculation and its outcome)

D. Molecular Method

E. Serology

Abortion

I. Etiologic agent ____________________

II. Classification

1	Domain	
2	Phylum	
3	Class	
4	Order	
5	Family	
6	Genus	

III. Sample Collection (from live and dead animal)

IV. Laboratory diagnosis

A) Direct Examination of the Specimen

B) Isolation and Identification of the agent

C) Pathogenicity test

D) Molecular Identification

E) Serology

A) Direct Examination of the Specimen

i) Staining method

Morphology by staining

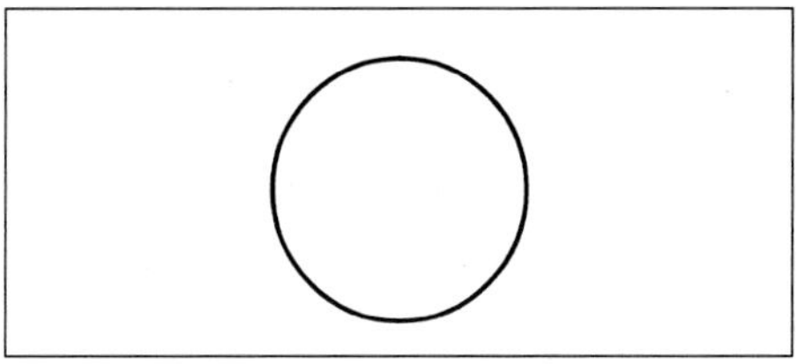

ii) Immunological method

iii) Nucleic acid method by direct sample

B) Isolation and Identification of the agent

i) Isolation of the agent

1. Basal/Enriched media ____________________

2. Selective/Differential media ____________________

ii) Identification of the agent

1. Staining method ____________________

Morphology

____

____

____

____

____

2. Colony characteristics in media

SOLID MEDIUM		**LIQUID MEDIUM**	
Shape		Degree of growth	
Size		Turbidity	
Elevation		Surface growth	
Surface		Odour	
Edge			
Opacity			
Colour			
Emulsifiability			

Growth in Media

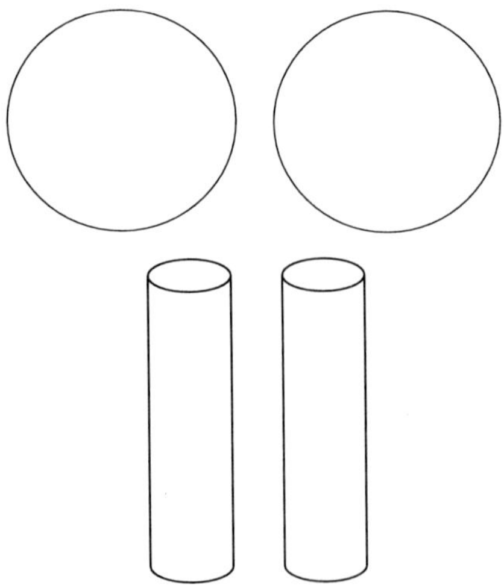

3. Biochemical characteristics

CARBOHYDRATE FERMENTATION TEST			
Arabinose		Inuline	
Dextrin		Mannose	
Dulcitol		Mannitol	
Fructose		Maltose	
Glucose		Salicin	
Glycerol		Sorbitol	
OTHER BIOCHEMICAL TEST			
Indole		Urease	
Methyl Red		H_2S production	
Voges Proskaur		Aesculine Hydrolysis	
Citrate			
Catalase			
Oxidase			
Nitrate			

4. Immunological/Antigen detection (Serotyping)

5. Nucleic acid method

C. Pathogenicity test - Animal Inoculation (name of the lab animal, route of inoculation and its outcome)

D. Molecular Method

E. Serology

Abortion

I. Etiologic agent ______________________________

II. Classification

1	Domain	
2	Phylum	
3	Class	
4	Order	
5	Family	
6	Genus	

III. Sample Collection (from live and dead animal)

____

____

____

____

IV. Laboratory diagnosis

A) Direct Examination of the Specimen

B) Isolation and Identification of the agent

C) Pathogenicity test

D) Molecular Identification

E) Serology

A) Direct Examination of the Specimen

i) Staining method

____

____

____

____

Morphology by staining

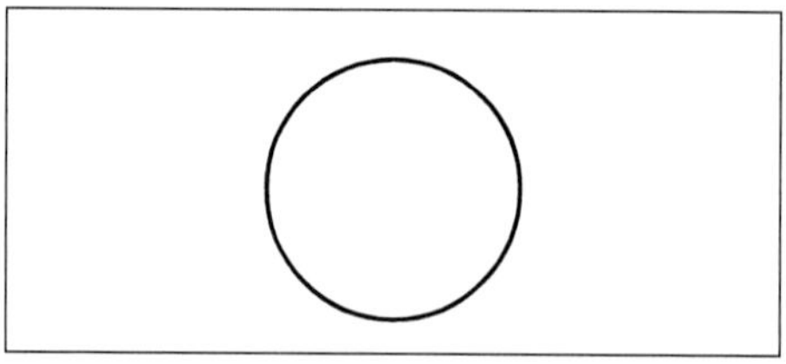

ii) Immunological method

iii) Nucleic acid method by direct sample

B) Isolation and Identification of the agent

i) Isolation of the agent –

1. Basal/Enriched media ______________________
2. Selective/Differential media ______________________

ii) Identification of the agent

1. Staining method ______________________

Morphology

2. Colony characteristics in media

SOLID MEDIUM		LIQUID MEDIUM	
Shape		Degree of growth	
Size		Turbidity	
Elevation		Surface growth	
Surface		Odour	
Edge			
Opacity			
Colour			
Emulsifiability			

Growth in Media

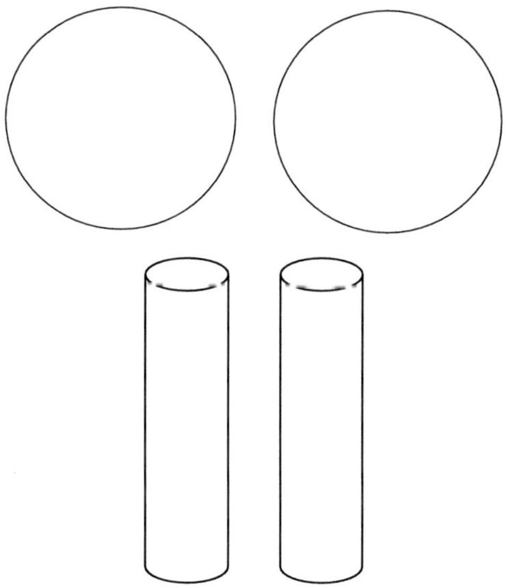

3. Biochemical characteristics

CARBOHYDRATE FERMENTATION TEST			
Arabinose		Inuline	
Dextrin		Mannose	
Dulcitol		Mannitol	
Fructose		Maltose	
Glucose		Salicin	
Glycerol		Sorbitol	
OTHER BIOCHEMICAL TEST			
Indole		Urease	
Methyl Red		H_2S production	
Voges Proskaur		Aesculine Hydrolysis	
Citrate			
Catalase			
Oxidase			
Nitrate			

4. Immunological/Antigen detection (Serotyping)

5. Nucleic acid method

C. Pathogenicity test - Animal Inoculation (name of the lab animal, route of inoculation and its outcome)

D. Molecular Method

E. Serology

Abortion

I. Etiologic agent ______________________________

II. Classification

1	Domain	
2	Phylum	
3	Class	
4	Order	
5	Family	
6	Genus	

III. Sample Collection (from live and dead animal)

____
____
____
____
____
____

IV. Laboratory diagnosis

A) Direct Examination of the Specimen

B) Isolation and Identification of the agent

C) Pathogenicity test

D) Molecular Identification

E) Serology

A) Direct Examination of the Specimen

i) Staining method

____
____
____
____
____

Morphology by staining

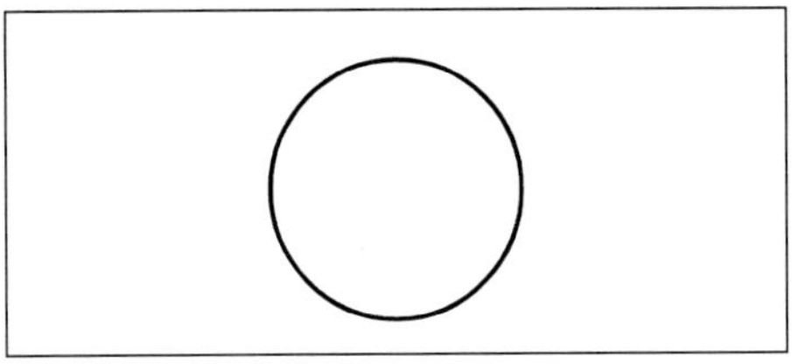

ii) Immunological method

iii) Nucleic acid method by direct sample

B) Isolation and Identification of the agent

i) Isolation of the agent

1. Basal/Enriched media ____________________

2. Selective/Differential media ____________________

ii) Identification of the agent

1. Staining method ____________________

Morphology

____

____

____

____

____

2. Colony characteristics in media

SOLID MEDIUM		**LIQUID MEDIUM**	
Shape		Degree of growth	
Size		Turbidity	
Elevation		Surface growth	
Surface		Odour	
Edge			
Opacity			
Colour			
Emulsifiability			

Growth in Media

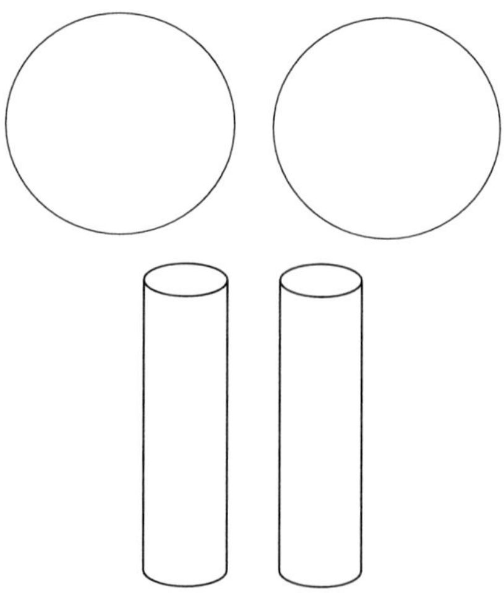

3. Biochemical characteristics

CARBOHYDRATE FERMENTATION TEST			
Arabinose		Inuline	
Dextrin		Mannose	
Dulcitol		Mannitol	
Fructose		Maltose	
Glucose		Salicin	
Glycerol		Sorbitol	
OTHER BIOCHEMICAL TEST			
Indole		Urease	
Methyl Red		H_2S production	
Voges Proskaur		Aesculine Hydrolysis	
Citrate			
Catalase			
Oxidase			
Nitrate			

4. Immunological/Antigen detection (Serotyping)

____

____

____

____

____

5. Nucleic acid method

____

____

____

____

____

C. Pathogenicity test - Animal Inoculation (name of the lab animal, route of inoculation and its outcome)

D. Molecular Method

E. Serology

Enteric

I. Etiologic agent ____________________

II. Classification

1	Domain	
2	Phylum	
3	Class	
4	Order	
5	Family	
6	Genus	

III. Sample Collection (from live and dead animal)

IV. Laboratory diagnosis

A) Direct Examination of the Specimen

B) Isolation and Identification of the agent

C) Pathogenicity test

D) Molecular Identification

E) Serology

A) Direct Examination of the Specimen

i) Staining method

Morphology by staining

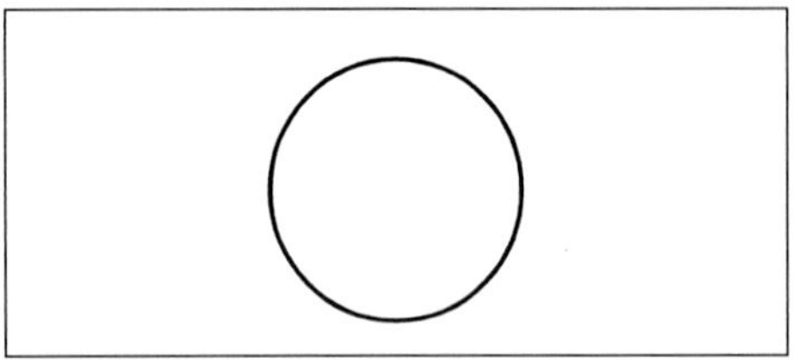

ii) Immunological method

iii) Nucleic acid method by direct sample

B) Isolation and Identification of the agent

i) Isolation of the agent

1. Basal/Enriched media ______________________

2. Selective/Differential media ______________________

ii) Identification of the agent

1. Staining method ______________________

Morphology

2. Colony characteristics in media

SOLID MEDIUM		LIQUID MEDIUM	
Shape		Degree of growth	
Size		Turbidity	
Elevation		Surface growth	
Surface		Odour	
Edge			
Opacity			
Colour			
Emulsifiability			

Growth in Media

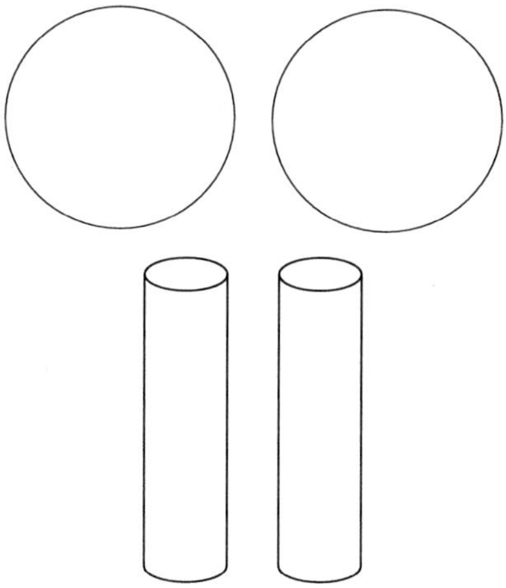

3. Biochemical characteristics

CARBOHYDRATE FERMENTATION TEST			
Arabinose		Inuline	
Dextrin		Mannose	
Dulcitol		Mannitol	
Fructose		Maltose	
Glucose		Salicin	
Glycerol		Sorbitol	
OTHER BIOCHEMICAL TEST			
Indole		Urease	
Methyl Red		H_2S production	
Voges Proskaur		Aesculine Hydrolysis	
Citrate			
Catalase			
Oxidase			
Nitrate			

4. Immunological/Antigen detection (Serotyping)

5. Nucleic acid method

C. Pathogenicity test - Animal Inoculation (name of the lab animal, route of inoculation and its outcome)

D. Molccular Method

E. Serology

Enteric

I. Etiologic agent ________________

II. Classification

1	Domain	
2	Phylum	
3	Class	
4	Order	
5	Family	
6	Genus	

III. Sample Collection (from live and dead animal)

____

____

____

____

____

IV. Laboratory diagnosis

A) Direct Examination of the Specimen

B) Isolation and Identification of the agent

C) Pathogenicity test

D) Molecular Identification

E) Serology

A) Direct Examination of the Specimen

i) Staining method

____

____

____

____

____

Morphology by staining

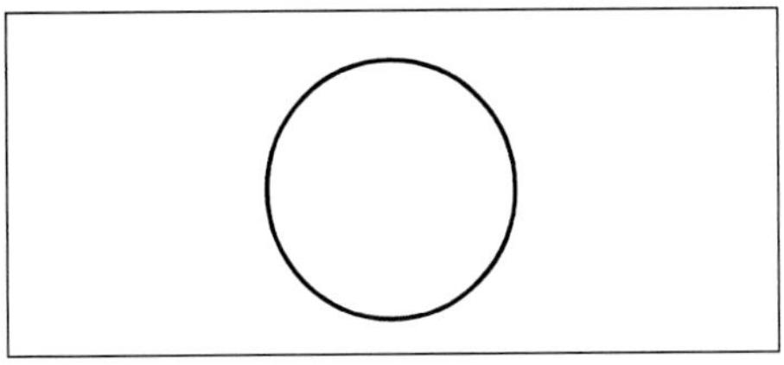

ii) Immunological method

____

____

____

____

____

iii) Nucleic acid method by direct sample

____

____

____

____

____

B) Isolation and Identification of the agent

i) Isolation of the agent

1. Basal/Enriched media ______________________________

2. Selective/Differential media ______________________________

ii) Identification of the agent

1. Staining method ______________________________

Morphology

____

____

____

____

____

2. Colony characteristics in media

SOLID MEDIUM		**LIQUID MEDIUM**	
Shape		Degree of growth	
Size		Turbidity	
Elevation		Surface growth	
Surface		Odour	
Edge			
Opacity			
Colour			
Emulsifiability			

Growth in Media

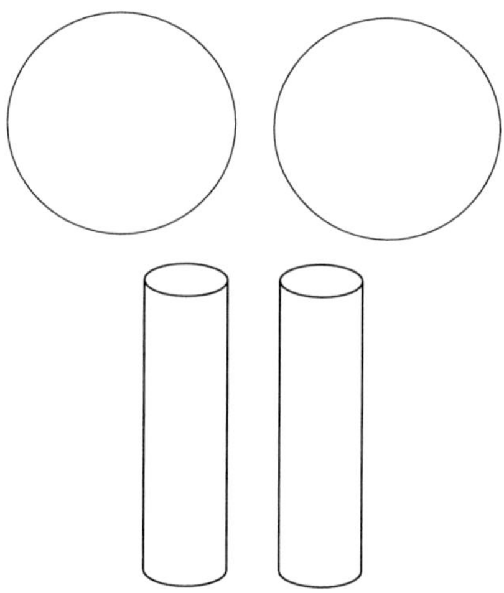

3. Biochemical characteristics

CARBOHYDRATE FERMENTATION TEST			
Arabinose		Inuline	
Dextrin		Mannose	
Dulcitol		Mannitol	
Fructose		Maltose	
Glucose		Salicin	
Glycerol		Sorbitol	
OTHER BIOCHEMICAL TEST			
Indole		Urease	
Methyl Red		H_2S production	
Voges Proskaur		Aesculine Hydrolysis	
Citrate			
Catalase			
Oxidase			
Nitrate			

4. Immunological/Antigen detection (Serotyping)

5. Nucleic acid method

C. Pathogenicity test - Animal Inoculation (name of the lab animal, route of inoculation and its outcome)

D. Molecular Method

E. Serology

Enteric

I. Etiologic agent ______

II. Classification

1	Domain	
2	Phylum	
3	Class	
4	Order	
5	Family	
6	Genus	

III. Sample Collection (from live and dead animal)

IV. Laboratory diagnosis

A) Direct Examination of the Specimen

B) Isolation and Identification of the agent

C) Pathogenicity test

D) Molecular Identification

E) Serology

A) Direct Examination of the Specimen:

i) Staining method

Morphology by staining

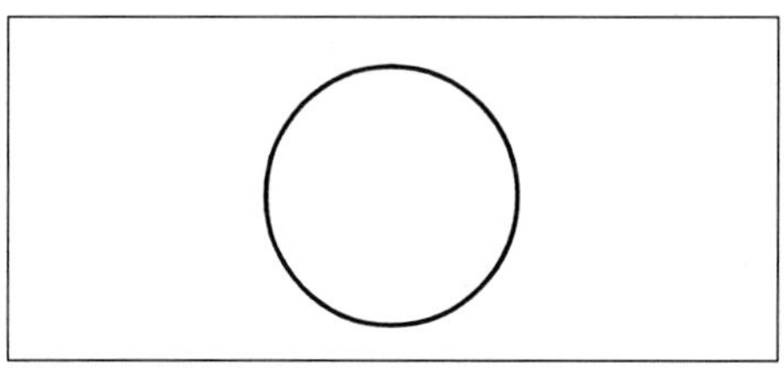

ii) Immunological method

iii) Nucleic acid method by direct sample

____

____

____

____

____

B) Isolation and Identification of the agent

i) Isolation of the agent

1. Basal/Enriched media ______________________

2. Selective/Differential media ______________________

ii) Identification of the agent

1. Staining method ______________________

Morphology

____

____

____

____

____

2. Colony characteristics in media

SOLID MEDIUM		LIQUID MEDIUM	
Shape		Degree of growth	
Size		Turbidity	
Elevation		Surface growth	
Surface		Odour	
Edge			
Opacity			
Colour			
Emulsifiability			

Growth in Media

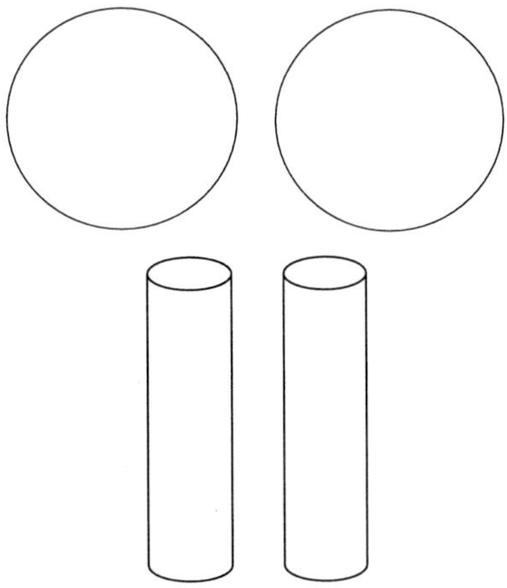

3. Biochemical characteristics

CARBOHYDRATE FERMENTATION TEST			
Arabinose		Inuline	
Dextrin		Mannose	
Dulcitol		Mannitol	
Fructose		Maltose	
Glucose		Salicin	
Glycerol		Sorbitol	
OTHER BIOCHEMICAL TEST			
Indole		Urease	
Methyl Red		H_2S production	
Voges Proskaur		Aesculine Hydrolysis	
Citrate			
Catalase			
Oxidase			
Nitrate			

4. Immunological/Antigen detection (Serotyping)

5. Nucleic acid method

C. Pathogenicity test - Animal Inoculation (name of the lab animal, route of inoculation and its outcome)

D. Molecular Method

E. Serology

Respiratory

I. Etiologic agent ___________________________

II. Classification

1	Domain	
2	Phylum	
3	Class	
4	Order	
5	Family	
6	Genus	

III. Sample Collection (from live and dead animal)

____

____

____

____

____

____

IV. Laboratory diagnosis

A) Direct Examination of the Specimen

B) Isolation and Identification of the agent

C) Pathogenicity test

D) Molecular Identification

E) Serology

A) Direct Examination of the Specimen

i) Staining method

____

____

____

____

____

____

Morphology by staining

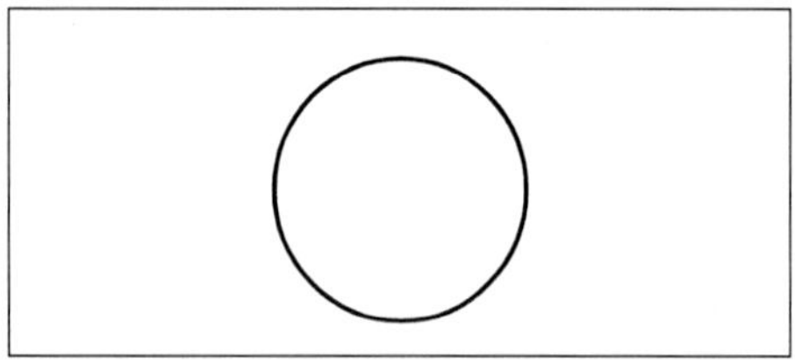

ii) Immunological method

iii) Nucleic acid method by direct sample

B) Isolation and Identification of the agent

i) Isolation of the agent

1. Basal/Enriched media ______________________

2. Selective/Differential media ______________________

ii) Identification of the agent

1. Staining method ______________________

Morphology

2. Colony characteristics in media

SOLID MEDIUM		LIQUID MEDIUM	
Shape		Degree of growth	
Size		Turbidity	
Elevation		Surface growth	
Surface		Odour	
Edge			
Opacity			
Colour			
Emulsifiability			

Growth in Media

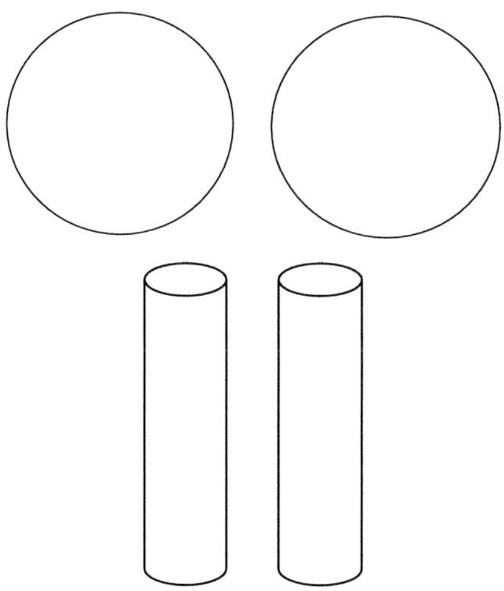

3. Biochemical characteristics

CARBOHYDRATE FERMENTATION TEST			
Arabinose		Inuline	
Dextrin		Mannose	
Dulcitol		Mannitol	
Fructose		Maltose	
Glucose		Salicin	
Glycerol		Sorbitol	
OTHER BIOCHEMICAL TEST			
Indole		Urease	
Methyl Red		H_2S production	
Voges Proskaur		Aesculine Hydrolysis	
Citrate			
Catalase			
Oxidase			
Nitrate			

4. Immunological/Antigen detection (Serotyping)

5. Nucleic acid method

C. Pathogenicity test - Animal Inoculation (name of the lab animal, route of inoculation and its outcome)

D. Molecular Method

E. Serology

Respiratory

I. Etiologic agent ______________________________

II. Classification

1	Domain	
2	Phylum	
3	Class	
4	Order	
5	Family	
6	Genus	

III. Sample Collection (from live and dead animal)

____

____

____

____

____

IV. Laboratory diagnosis

A) Direct Examination of the Specimen

B) Isolation and Identification of the agent

C) Pathogenicity test

D) Molecular Identification

E) Serology

A) Direct Examination of the Specimen

i) Staining method

____

____

____

____

____

Morphology by staining

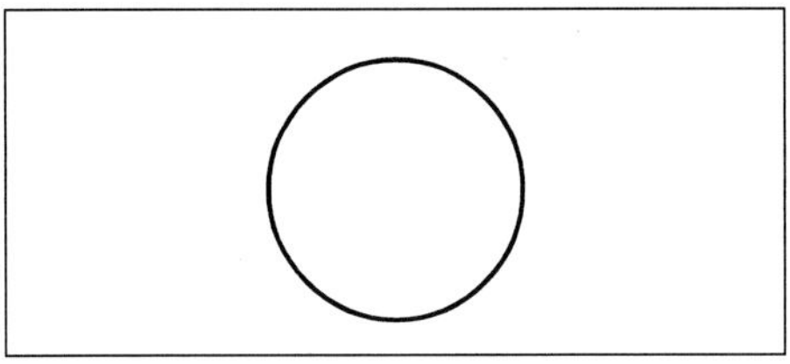

ii) Immunological method

iii) Nucleic acid method by direct sample

B) Isolation and Identification of the agent

i) Isolation of the agent –

1. Basal/Enriched media ____________________

2. Selective/Differential media ____________________

ii) Identification of the agent

1. Staining method ____________________

Morphology

2. Colony characteristics in media

SOLID MEDIUM		**LIQUID MEDIUM**	
Shape		Degree of growth	
Size		Turbidity	
Elevation		Surface growth	
Surface		Odour	
Edge			
Opacity			
Colour			
Emulsifiability			

Growth in Media

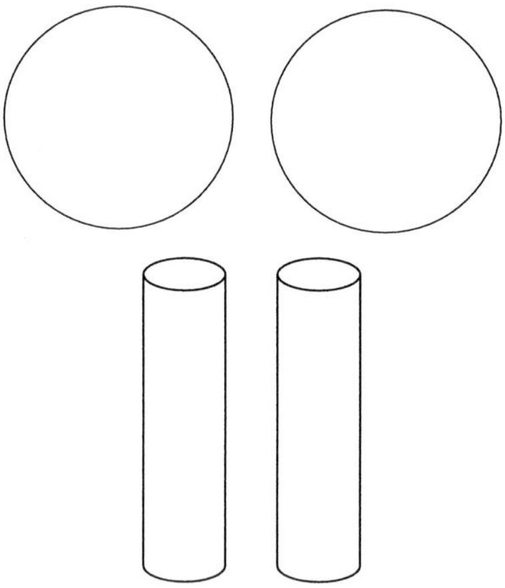

3. Biochemical characteristics

CARBOHYDRATE FERMENTATION TEST			
Arabinose		Inuline	
Dextrin		Mannose	
Dulcitol		Mannitol	
Fructose		Maltose	
Glucose		Salicin	
Glycerol		Sorbitol	
OTHER BIOCHEMICAL TEST			
Indole		Urease	
Methyl Red		H_2S production	
Voges Proskaur		Aesculine Hydrolysis	
Citrate			
Catalase			
Oxidase			
Nitrate			

4. Immunological/Antigen detection (Serotyping)

5. Nucleic acid method

C. Pathogenicity test - Animal Inoculation (name of the lab animal, route of inoculation and its outcome)

D. Molecular Method

E. Serology

Pyogenic infections

I. Etiologic agent ______________________________

II. Classification

1	Domain	
2	Phylum	
3	Class	
4	Order	
5	Family	
6	Genus	

III. Sample Collection (from live and dead animal)

____

____

____

____

____

IV. Laboratory diagnosis

A) Direct Examination of the Specimen

B) Isolation and Identification of the agent

C) Pathogenicity test

D) Molecular Identification

E) Serology

A) Direct Examination of the Specimen

i) Staining method

____

____

____

____

____

Morphology by staining

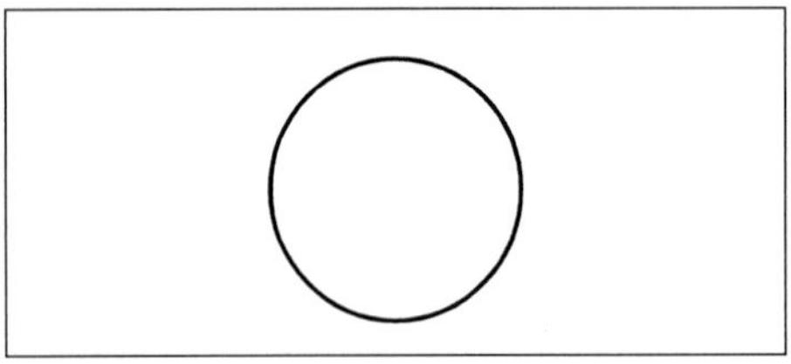

ii) Immunological method

iii) Nucleic acid method by direct sample

B) Isolation and Identification of the agent

i) Isolation of the agent

1. Basal/Enriched media ______________________

2. Selective/Differential media ______________________

ii) Identification of the agent

1. Staining method ______________________

Morphology

____

____

____

____

____

2. Colony characteristics in media

SOLID MEDIUM		**LIQUID MEDIUM**	
Shape		Degree of growth	
Size		Turbidity	
Elevation		Surface growth	
Surface		Odour	
Edge			
Opacity			
Colour			
Emulsifiability			

Growth in Media

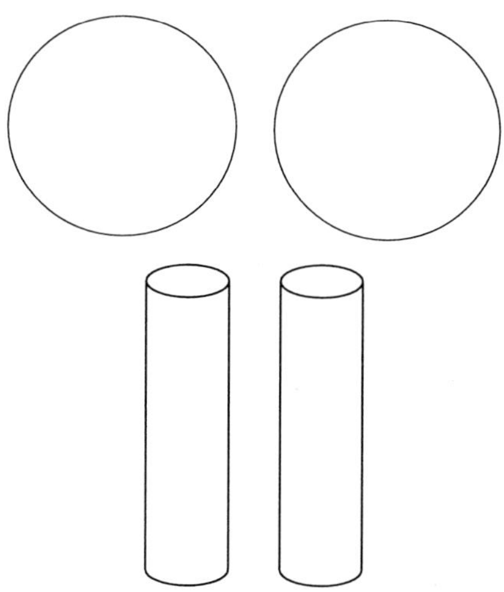

3. Biochemical characteristics

CARBOHYDRATE FERMENTATION TEST			
Arabinose		Inuline	
Dextrin		Mannose	
Dulcitol		Mannitol	
Fructose		Maltose	
Glucose		Salicin	
Glycerol		Sorbitol	
OTHER BIOCHEMICAL TEST			
Indole		Urease	
Methyl Red		H_2S production	
Voges Proskaur		Aesculine Hydrolysis	
Citrate			
Catalase			
Oxidase			
Nitrate			

4. Immunological/Antigen detection (Serotyping)

5. Nucleic acid method

C. Pathogenicity test - Animal Inoculation (name of the lab animal, route of inoculation and its outcome)

D. Molecular Method

E. Serology

Pyogenic infections

I. Etiologic agent ____________________

II. Classification

1	Domain	
2	Phylum	
3	Class	
4	Order	
5	Family	
6	Genus	

III. Sample Collection (from live and dead animal)

IV. Laboratory diagnosis

A) Direct Examination of the Specimen
B) Isolation and Identification of the agent
C) Pathogenicity test
D) Molecular Identification
E) Serology

A) Direct Examination of the Specimen

i) Staining method

Morphology by staining

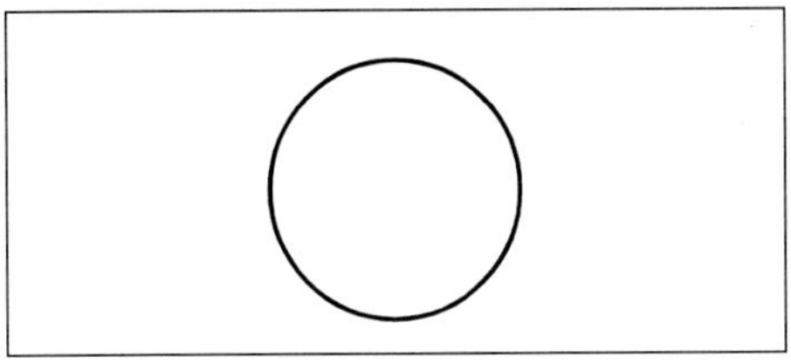

ii) Immunological method

iii) Nucleic acid method by direct sample

B) Isolation and Identification of the agent

i) Isolation of the agent

1. Basal/Enriched media ______

2. Selective/Differential media ______

ii) Identification of the agent

1. Staining method ______

Morphology

2. Colony characteristics in media

SOLID MEDIUM		LIQUID MEDIUM	
Shape		Degree of growth	
Size		Turbidity	
Elevation		Surface growth	
Surface		Odour	
Edge			
Opacity			
Colour			
Emulsifiability			

Growth in Media

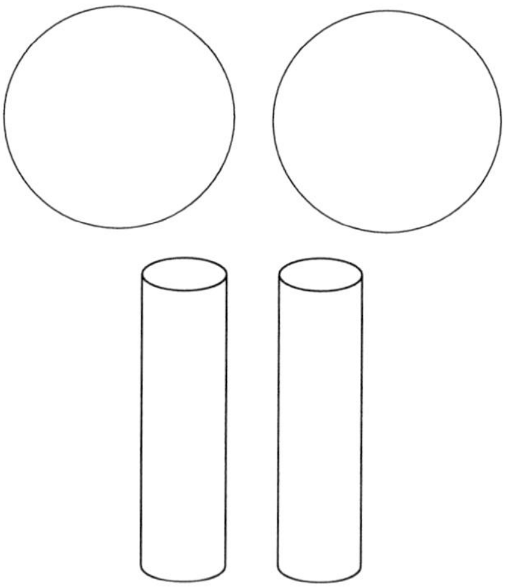

3. Biochemical characteristics

CARBOHYDRATE FERMENTATION TEST			
Arabinose		Inuline	
Dextrin		Mannose	
Dulcitol		Mannitol	
Fructose		Maltose	
Glucose		Salicin	
Glycerol		Sorbitol	
OTHER BIOCHEMICAL TEST			
Indole		Urease	
Methyl Red		H_2S production	
Voges Proskaur		Aesculine Hydrolysis	
Citrate			
Catalase			
Oxidase			
Nitrate			

4. Immunological/Antigen detection (Serotyping)

5. Nucleic acid method

C. Pathogenicity test - Animal Inoculation (name of the lab animal, route of inoculation and its outcome)

D. Molecular Method

E. Serology

Pyogenic infections

I. Etiologic agent ____________________

II. Classification

1	Domain	
2	Phylum	
3	Class	
4	Order	
5	Family	
6	Genus	

III. Sample Collection (from live and dead animal)

IV. Laboratory diagnosis

A) Direct Examination of the Specimen
B) Isolation and Identification of the agent
C) Pathogenicity test
D) Molecular Identification
E) Serology

A) Direct Examination of the Specimen

i) Staining method

Morphology by staining

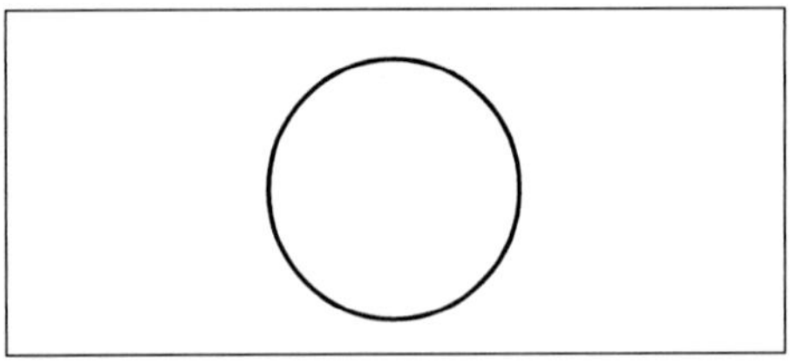

ii) Immunological method

iii) Nucleic acid method by direct sample

B) Isolation and Identification of the agent

i) Isolation of the agent

1. Basal/Enriched media ____________________

2. Selective/Differential media ____________________

ii) Identification of the agent

1. Staining method ____________________

Morphology

2. Colony characteristics in media

SOLID MEDIUM		**LIQUID MEDIUM**	
Shape		Degree of growth	
Size		Turbidity	
Elevation		Surface growth	
Surface		Odour	
Edge			
Opacity			
Colour			
Emulsifiability			

Growth in Media

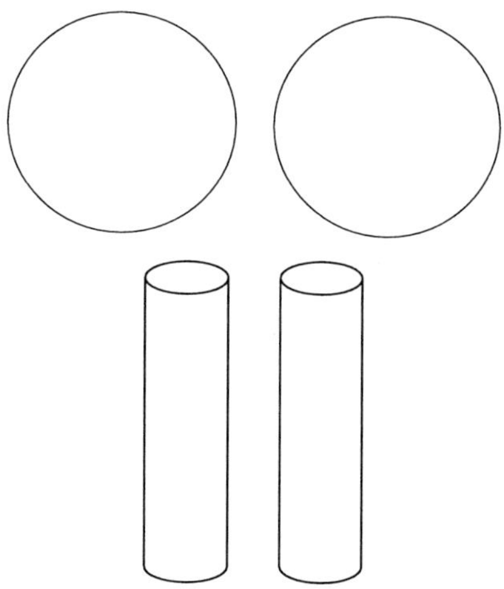

3. Biochemical characteristics

CARBOHYDRATE FERMENTATION TEST			
Arabinose		Inuline	
Dextrin		Mannose	
Dulcitol		Mannitol	
Fructose		Maltose	
Glucose		Salicin	
Glycerol		Sorbitol	
OTHER BIOCHEMICAL TEST			
Indole		Urease	
Methyl Red		H_2S production	
Voges Proskaur		Aesculine Hydrolysis	
Citrate			
Catalase			
Oxidase			
Nitrate			

4. Immunological/Antigen detection (Serotyping)

5. Nucleic acid method

C. Pathogenicity test - Animal Inoculation (name of the lab animal, route of inoculation and its outcome)

D. Molecular Method

E. Serology